Hope This Meets You In Good Health

Prahlādānanda Swami

To His Divine Grace A. C. Bhaktivedanta Swami Prabhupāda,
my eternal guide and master who opened my eyes with spiritual
and material awareness.

Table of Contents

Foreword 9

Preface 13

Introduction 15

Chapter 1 General Principles for Health 19

1. Health Comes First 19
2. Take Care of Kṛṣṇa's Body 21
3. Healthy Life or Self-Preservation 24
4. Kṛṣṇa's Service Comes First 25
5. Protect the Body 30
6. Regulation in Habits and Simple Eating 31
   i. Prabhupāda's Daily Schedule 33
   ii. Gurukula Schedule 34
7. Teach Them Not to Fall Sick 36
8. Don't Misuse the Body, Use It for Freedom 37
9. Pure Mind and Hygienic in Body 39
10. Best Use of a Bad Bargain 39
11. Old House 43
12. Not Too Cold 45
13. Tolerance 45
14. Temple of Disease 47
15. Woman's Health and Having Children 48
16. Don't Leave Remnants of Food 48
17. Duties in Relation to the Body and Mind 50
18. Don't Bother Very Much with the Body 51

Chapter 2 Health and Sickness in Spiritual Life 52

19. Everything Depends on Kṛṣṇa 52
20. Work on the Spiritual Platform 53
21. Real Healthy Life is Kṛṣṇa Consciousness 54
22. Spiritual Advancement Will Keep the Body Healthy 54
23. Relief from Bodily and Spiritual Diseases 62
24. Real Hospital 64
25. Devotees Should Look After the Other Devotees 65
    i. Ask Them What They Need 65
    ii. GBC's Concern 66
    iii. Sympathetic 67

Chapter 3 Maintaining Health 69

26. Diet 69
    i. Basis of All Food 69
    ii. Diet for a Sick Devotee 71
    iii. Eat Nice Nutritious Food 72
    iv. Raw Diet 72
    v. *Prasāda* and Preaching 73
    vi. Eat Only Prasāda, Food Offered to Lord Kṛṣṇa 74
    vii. Tapasya and Detachment 76
27. Foods and Herbs and Spices 83
    i. Aloe Vera and Garlic 83
    ii. Boysenberries 84
    iii. Castor Seeds 84
    iv. Chili 85
    v. Chickpeas 85
    vi. Iron Pills 86
    vii. Nima (Neem) 86
    viii. Ghee 86
    ix. Mangoes 87
    x. Milk for Expecting Mothers 87
    xi. Milk is Nectar 88

xii. Milk and Halavā 89
xiii. Milk and Salt 89
xiv. Yogurt 89
xv. Dried – Banana Chips 89
xvi. Rice, *Dāl*, and Chapattis, etc. 90
xvii. Puffed Rice 90
xviii. Spices 91
xix. Watermelon 92
xx. Water 93
xxi. Undesirable Food 94
28. Cleanliness 97
29. Exercise 99
i. Too Much Not Necessary 99
ii. Swimming and Bathing in the Ocean 99
iii. Wake Up Early and Morning Walks 100
iv. Yoga 102
30. Massage and Other Things 107
31. Climate 108
32. Sleeping 108
33. Toothbrush 109
34. Mental Health 109
i. Mental Health—Psychiatry 109

Chapter 4 Treating Disease 114

35. Treat the Root Cause 114
36. Bad Signs 114
37. Birth, Death, Old Age, and Disease 115
38. Natural Life 118
39. Holy Place 118
40. Consult Approved Physician 119
41. Control the Discharge of Semen 119
42. Deafness 120
43. Doctors 120
44. Dispensary 122

45. The Holy Names 123
46. Take Rest If Sick 124
47. Proper and Practical 126
48. Illness and Remedies 126
i. Ailment of the Finger 126
ii. Antiseptic 126
iii. Appetite 127
iv. Asthma 127
v. Bleeding 128
vi. Cancer 128
vii. Childbirth 128
viii. Colds 129
ix. Conception 129
x. Diarrhea 129
xi. Dry Skin 129
xii. Dysentery 129
xiii. Headache 130
xiv. Heat Stroke 130
xv. High Fever 130
xvi. Infection 131
xvii. Intestines and Arteries 131
xviii. Irregularity in Hunger and Thirst 131
xix. Jaundice and Liver Disease 132
xx. Nervous Instability 134
xxi. Rheumatism 135
xxii. Sore Throat 136
xxiii. Syphilis and Venereal Disease 136
xxiv. Toothache 137
xxv. Whooping Cough 138
xxvi. Worms 138
49. Quick Treatment 138
50. Kinds of Treatments 139
i. Āyurveda 139
ii. Homeopathic Medicine 149

iii. Massage 150
iv. Medicine 151
v. Nature Cure 154
vi. Pilly Consciousness 154
vii. Surgery 154
viii. Vaccines 157

Chapter 5 Some Amazing Stories from the Scriptures 159

51. Hiraṇyakaśipu and Lord Brahmā 159
52. Indra and His Elephant 162
53. Sanātana Gosvāmī and Itching Sores 163
54. The Leper Vāsudeva and Lord Caitanya 164
55. Śrīvāsa Ṭhākura's Son Dies 165
56. Sāraṅga Ṭhākura and Murāri Caitanya dāsa 166
57. Prahlāda Mahārāja Fed Poison 166
58. Cyavana Muni 166

The Hunchback Kubja Becomes Beautiful 167

Chapter 6 Articles on Health by Prahlādānanda Swami 177

59. Āyurveda 101 177
60. Āyurveda 102 180
61. Āyurveda 103 188
62. The Four Pillars of Treatment 193
63. Reduction and Tonification 197
64. Some Hints to Keep Healthy 201
65. Routine, a Secret of Health 206
66. Sadhana and Health 210
67. Rules for Enlightenment and Happiness 213
68. Yama and Niyama 213
69. Pranayama 221
70. Celibacy 227

Foreword

Āyurveda is an ancient system of healing the body, mind, and consciousness. In the true sense of the word, Ayurveda hugs the whole person. Ayurveda has its root in the Vedic literature, both the Rig Veda and the Atharva Veda.

Āyurveda says that every human being is a unique expression of the cosmos. *Purushoyam loka sammitah ayam purushah loka sammitah. Loka* means "universe," and *sammita* means "collection," so every human being is a collection of the basic principles of the universe. In other words, every conscious being (*purusha*) is a combination of primordial matter (*prakriti*), cosmic intelligence (*mahat*), and ego, the feeling of "I am" (*ahankara*). So every individual is indivisible, i.e., an undivided, total, unique expression of the cosmos. Therefore, that individual approach is there in Āyurveda – Āyurveda is individualistic healing, individualistic medicine. Prahlādānanda Swami has beautifully explained these principles of Āyurveda in his wonderful book *Hope This Meets You in Good Health*. This is a practical guide that will enable anyone to adopt Ayurvedic principles in his or her life to heal the body, the mind, and the consciousness.

Ether, air, fire, water, and earth are the further expression of consciousness. Ether, nuclear energy, is present in every cell, tissue, and organ system. All cavities in the body are space, or ether. There is abdominal space, thoracic space, cranial space; every space is a system. So it is a spacious system, which is called srotas. Srotas is a channel, and the body is made up of many, many srotamsi. In that srotas akash, the space is there. Between two cells there is a space, called intercellular space, and in that intercellular space one cell communicates with another. So cellular communication is possible because of space.

Then there is movement, which is sensory stimuli, motor responsive. Our lungs are breathing, which is movement, our diaphragm is moving up and down, which is movement, our heart is beating, which is movement, and there are subtle gastrointestinal movement, uterine movement, movement in the fallopian tube, movement within the ovaries and testicles. All these bodily movements are governed by the element air – the wind, prana.

Where there is movement there is friction, and where there is friction there is heat, agni. Agni is body temperature, agni is digestive enzymes, agni is nothing but the process of digestion, absorption, assimilation, and transformation of food into constituents the body can use. Therefore agni governs metabolic activities in the body.

The fourth element is water. Water is plasma, serum, cytoplasm; water is saliva, sweat, urine; and water is present in the cerebrospinal fluid. Without water, there is no nutrition. So bodily water is constantly lubricating and hydrating the bodily cells.

Then, finally, comes earth. All organic and inorganic matter is made up of five great elements – calcium, magnesium, zinc, copper, and iron. All these elements are present in the bones, in the cartilage, in the hair, in the teeth. So the human body is made up of five great elements. This is the structural aspect of the human body.

The functional aspect of the human body is further grouped into three biological combinations of ether, air, fire, water, and earth. The combination of ether and air constitute vata dosa, which is a principle of movement. Fire and water constitute pitta dosa, which is the energy of transformation. And kapha dosa is the combination of water and earth. Kapha is necessary for building-block material. Vata, pitta, kapha – these three constituents are present in the body of everyone. At the time of making love, whatever dosa is predominant in the body, mind, and consciousness of the father and mother will determine the constitution of the child. For example, at the time of fertilization if the father has excess pitta and the mother has excess kapha, then the baby will have a pitta/kapha constitution.

Now, a unique combination of vata, pitta, and kapha are present in every human being according to one's unique prakriti, or constitution. Prakriti doesn't change, but bodily dosas do change because of changes in age, diet, weather, atmosphere, relationships, etc. This changing status of the dosas is called vikriti. So, prakriti/vikriti is the basic paradigm of this book by Prahlādānanda Swami, *Hope This Meets You in Good Health.* This book is a practical guide. He gives us very simple instructions to control the dosas and deal with asthma, cancer, arthritis, rheumatism, sciatica, and other ailments. He gives very practical guidance to the reader.

Prahlādānanda Swami is a very senior and intimate disciple of Śrīla Prabhupāda, the founder and spiritual guide of the Hare Krishna movement. Prabhupāda was a highly enlightened master. He was a great yogi, but he never claimed that he was a great yogi. The way he walked, the way he talked – he was perfectly spiritual. In this book Prahlādānanda Swami has given a detailed description of Srila Prabhupāda's daily routine. If you follow the diet and daily routine that Prabhupāda followed, your life will radically change for the better. In other words, you will attain perfect health – physical, mental, and spiritual.

I hope that this book will guide you in every step of your life.

Hare Krishna.

Dr. Vasant Lad

Preface

For decades Prahlādānanda Swami has been a caring educator and an inspiring example of the benefits of natural healing. Ever since I met him in Śrīdhāma Māyāpur in the nineties, he has supported my natural health service with infinite grace.

The spiritual perspective devotees have on disease is a revelation to me. They accept illness as a positive purification, a reminder that the body is fallible and the soul infallible. I've seen devotees even embrace sickness as a spiritual lesson and accept it as the consequence of their actions; they valued the opportunity to 'burn off their karma.' Adversity gave rise to insight, empathy, and an appreciation of blessings.

Śrīla Prabhupāda had the same practical and philosophical approach. Illness is inevitable, but to some extent how much we suffer depends on our perception and expectations. Srila Prabhupāda taught us to live prudently and maintain a healthy diet and a good balance between rest, exercise, and spiritual practices. He combined home herbal remedies with Āyurvedic expertise that often alleviated suffering. His daily diet and routine incorporated healing touches, such as massage and ginger lemon appetizers. But ultimately Srila Prabhupāda advised us not to obsess about health, for the body is a tool for service and not for unhealthy sense gratification. And if our bodies break down, we can spiritually progress by accessing our immortal, invincible soul. As Prabhupāda said, a "healthy life is to become God conscious." (Conversation, London, July 11, 1973)

The wonderful wisdom in this book can bestow upon its readers better health. Since the book is also a tool to assist others, I pray many will benefit from its timeless truths. And, of course, I hope this meets you all in good health!

Rāga Maṇjarī Devī Dāsī (Caroline Robertson)
Naturopath, Homoeopath, Āyurvedic consultant

Introduction

Maintaining good health has always been part of my life. In my childhood my family thought that eating only fruits one day a week would be healthful, but we couldn't follow such a diet for long. My mother believed that natural cures were more efficacious than allopathic ones, and thus our family's primary health-care provider was a chiropractor. In my school days, especially during high school, I played many sports, for exercise was important to me. And before joining the International Society for Krishna Consciousness (ISKCON) in 1968, I studied *haṭha-yoga*. Nowadays, apart from regularly practicing this kind of *yoga* (I've recently become a certified Iyengar yoga teacher), I practice Tai Chi Chaun and study astrology (*jyotiṣa*) from a medical perspective.

I joined the Kṛṣṇa consciousness movement when I was nineteen, and whenever I had direct association with Śrīla Prabhupāda I observed his regulated diet and regular massages and sometimes accompanied him during his daily morning walks. In many of his letters, which he characteristically closed with "Hope this meets you in good health," he expressed his genuine concern for his disciples' health. His wisdom in dealing with his own illness and that of others was profound and obvious. All this clearly indicated to me that physical and mental health was something integral to Kṛṣṇa consciousness, or the path of devotion to the Supreme Lord, the method of spiritual realization I have been practicing for over four decades now.

In 1987 I was asked to teach a course on health at the Vṛndṛvana Institute for Higher Education (VIHE). After investigating Śrīla Prabhupāda's books, I concluded that it would be most appropriate for me to teach ISKCON devotees Āyurveda, the Vedic science of health. Thus I began consulting various Āyurvedic doctors and studying books on the ancient science of Āyurvedic healing. In the course of my devotional career I also became a member of the ISKCON Health and Welfare Committee, which later became the ISKCON Health and Welfare Ministry, of which I am now the Minister.

Once a year the Ministry publishes *Hope This Meets You in Good Health*, a magazine featuring articles about health issues written mostly by ISKCON members. Each magazine includes a section of quotes on health from Śrīla Prabhupāda's books, letters, lectures, etc., and from the previous *ācāryas* (spiritual teachers). Having published more than a dozen issues of the magazine, I am convinced that these valuable instructions on health should also be presented as a book. Hence this volume. To make the book more interesting and relevant, I have also included anecdotes taken from biographical accounts of Śrīla Prabhupāda written by his disciples, such as Satsvarūpa dāsa Gosvāmī and Hari Śauri Dāsa.

Although this book offers but a small drop from the ocean of health science, Śrīla Prabhupāda's instructions and personal example give all spiritual aspirants invaluable insights into how a devotee of Kṛṣṇa keeps good health. Śrīla Prabhupāda himself did so while simultaneously leading a demanding spiritual life of meditation on the Supreme Lord, teaching rigorously, and spreading the message of Kṛṣṇa consciousness all over the world.

Śrīla Prabhupāda's books, letters, and transcribed lectures generally include the Sanskrit diacritical marks, and they have been retained in the following pages. You'll find a guide to Sanskrit pronunciation on page 242. We briefly explain in the text the Sanskrit terms relevant to the book's main topic of health and welfare. Sanskrit terms not germane to the main topic are defined in the glossary. Since the quotations found in this book come from various sources, some inconsistencies in spelling may occur. For instance, *prasāda* and *prasādam* are alternate spellings for the Sanskrit word for sanctified food.

In addition, this book contains many names or phrases that refer to the Divinity, such as "Lord Kṛṣṇa," "Lord Viṣṇu," "The Supreme Personality of Godhead," and "the Absolute Truth." All these terms refer to the one Supreme Lord who is referred to as "God" in various cultures and languages.

When A. C. Bhaktivedanta Swami, affectionately known to his followers as Śrīla Prabhupāda, first arrived in America from India, he carried with him some Indian rupees (worth about twenty-four dollars) and two trunks. One was filled with the first three printed volumes of his still incomplete translation of the ancient religious and philosophical classic *Śrīmad-Bhāgavatam*; the second contained rolled wheat. And in the other trunk a large bundle of cereal that he could eat for breakfast.

Over the next twelve years Prabhupāda created a movement that started from nothing but grew to over five thousand devoted followers and a hundred temples around the world. Even among success stories his is astounding, but what makes it even more amazing is that when he arrived in the USA he was sixty-nine years old and had suffered two heart attacks on his grueling sea journey. And although he was at an advanced age and suffered from numerous illnesses, some because of old age and others because of constant travel to spread his movement, his vibrant energy still surpassed that of his youthful followers, who were in their teens or early twenties.

While a family man in India, Śrīla Prabhupāda gained some medical knowledge through his occupation as a pharmacist. He also possessed what could be called "granny" wisdom about health remedies that were common knowledge when he grew up. He applied this knowledge and wisdom in his life and also shared it, especially with his students and followers.

Although Śrīla Prabhupāda emphasized that we should all transcend material existence, he never minimized the value of good health, above all for those who have yet to transcend the soul's misidentification with the material body. But Śrīla Prabhupāda also never overemphasized health at the cost of spiritual advancement or serving the spiritual mission he had inherited from a line of teachers going back to Lord Caitanya Mahāprabhu, who is considered an incarnation of the Supreme Personality of Godhead, or God. Mahāprabhu's mission was to reveal absolute reality and show by His personal example how to lead a pure devotional life in service to God. As Śrīla Prabhupāda endeavored to fulfill that mission, he had to balance his spiritual endeavors with the need to work within the limitations of the material body. His personal behavior clearly showed that he succeeded in this, and his instructions were meant to help us attain the same balance. Thus those who appreciate or who are part of the mission Śrīla Prabhupāda expanded — and continues to expand — around the world will find these instructions most valuable, for they give a spiritual perspective on health along with practical advice on how to deal with various health problems.

Such a perspective and such advice will likely be appreciated even by readers unfamiliar with Śrīla Prabhupāda and his mission.

In a world in which birth, death, old age, and disease are all-pervading, Śrīla Prabhupāda, expertly judging time, place, and audience, placed more or less emphasis on health matters. Of course, he wanted his disciples to remain healthy, but he also wanted them to sincerely use their energy and resources in the service of the Supreme Lord without being unnecessarily distracted by bodily concerns. Usually Śrīla Prabhupāda found no conflict between health and devotional service, but at times he did, and in the first part of this book we explain how he dealt with such tensions and showed that they need not cause confusion. Rather, such tensions illustrate how under diverse circumstances different — indeed sometimes seemingly contradictory — solutions apply.

In short, Part One of this book attempts to offer insight into how a self-realized soul, an advanced transcendentalist beyond the bodily concept of life, dealt with both common and serious health issues and how he expected his followers to deal with them.

The second and final part of the book consists of articles I wrote for *Hope This Meets You in Good Health* and other publications. To be sure, I do not presume that these articles are in any way an exhaustive treatment of Āyurveda, but I hope that, as a compilation, they may serve as a brief introduction to this profound and valuable medical science.

Prahlādānanda Swami

Chapter 1
General Principles for Health

Health Comes First

Although the soul is transcendental to the material body, when conditioned by material nature, the soul's consciousness becomes affected by different material circumstances. Therefore, aspiring devotees should try to keep themselves in situations that are conducive to the steady and enthusiastic execution of devotional service. As Śrīla Prabhupāda writes:

When a living entity is conditioned, he has two kinds of activities: one is conditional, and the other is constitutional. As for protecting the body or abiding by the rules of society and state, certainly there are different activities, even for the devotees, in connection with the conditional life, and such activities are called conditional. Besides these, the living entity who is fully conscious of his spiritual nature and is engaged in Kṛṣṇa consciousness, or the devotional service of the Lord, has activities which are called transcendental. Such activities are performed in his constitutional position, and they are technically called devotional service. Now, in the conditioned state, sometimes devotional service and the conditional service in relation to the body will parallel one another. But then again, sometimes these activities become opposed to one another. As far as possible, a devotee is very cautious so that he does not do anything that could disrupt his wholesome condition. He knows that perfection in his activities depends on his progressive realization of Kṛṣṇa consciousness.

(Bhagavad-gītā 9.30, purport)

Be careful about your health first. This information is not only for you but for all my noble sons. I am an old man. I may live or die it does not matter. But you must live for a long time to push on this Kṛṣṇa consciousness movement.

(Letter to Rāyarāma Dāsa, December 21, 1967)

The first thing is that you must feel well. In whatever condition you should feel well, because if you fall sick, everything will be topsy-turvy. And what you require to be in good health, you know better than anyone else. That is your first business.

(Letter to Brahmānanda, May 15, 1969)

He [Kardama Muni] looked healthy because he had directly received the nectarean sound vibrations from the lotus lips of the Personality of Godhead. Similarly, one who hears the transcendental sound vibration of the holy name of the Lord, Hare Kṛṣṇa, also improves in health. We have actually seen that many *brahmacārīs* and *gṛhasthas* connected with the International Society for Kṛṣṇa consciousness have improved in health, and a luster has come to their faces. It is essential that a *brahmacārī* engaged in spiritual advancement look very healthy and lustrous.

(Śrīmad-Bhāgavatam 3.21.45-47, purport)

The soldiers in this Kṛṣṇa consciousness movement must always possess physical strength, enthusiasm, and sensual power. To keep themselves fit, they must therefore place themselves in a normal condition of life. What constitutes a normal condition will not be the same for everyone, and therefore there are divisions of varṇāśrama — *brāhmaṇa*, *kṣatriya*, *vaiśya*, *Śūdra*, *brahmacarya*, *gṛhastha*, *vānaprastha*, and *sannyasa*.

(Śrīmad-Bhāgavatam 8.2.30, purport)

I told Prabhupāda that Harikeśa thinks his condition is colitis. And he feels that if he stays in India, it will only get worse. He feels that only a return to the West will enable him to get well. But while he feels this way, Harikeśa just doesn't want to leave Prabhupāda's service. But Prabhupāda told me that one's health is primary.

(Transcendental Diary, Vol.1, Chap. 9, January 31, 1976)

Take Care of Kṛṣṇa's Body

Everything belongs to Lord Kṛṣṇa and is meant for His pleasure; this includes even the body of His devotees. Therefore, a devotee does not neglect his health, but tries to maintain it to keep the body fit for the service of the Supreme Lord. The devotee doesn't eat too much or too little, sleep too much or too little. He does what is necessary to optimize his devotional service.

So far Jadurāṇī is concerned, inform her that this body is Kṛṣṇa's body. Therefore, she should take care of her health. Of course it is very encouraging that she puts forward service of Kṛṣṇa first, then all other consideration. It is very nice, and I very much appreciate this attempt. But still, we should not neglect about our health. Because the body of a devotee is not material. The body of a devotee should not be neglected as material. This has been warned by the Goswāmīs, that we should not neglect any material thing if it can be used for Kṛṣṇa consciousness. So her body, because it is engaged in Kṛṣṇa's service, is valuable. So not only she, but all of you, should take care of this poor girl. She has left her parents and she is unmarried, no husband, so of course, she is not poor, because she has got so many God-brothers, and sisters, and above all Kṛṣṇa, she is not at all poor. In spite of that, we should care about her health. That is our duty, and inform her that she may not strain beyond her capacity. Of course, such kinds of trouble may come and go, a devotee is not afraid of such things, but still it is our duty to think always that this is Kṛṣṇa's body, and this must not be neglected.

(Letter to Satsvarūpa Dāsa, August 19, 1968)

Ugrakarma is intense work that is unhealthy and inauspicious

I am very much concerned about yourself, that you have been injured, by working. I do not know what sort of *ugrakarma* you were doing, but whatever you do, you must be careful. Your body is dedicated to Kṛṣṇa; therefore you should not be neglectful about your body. You should always think that your body is not more your body, but it is Kṛṣṇa's body. Therefore, you should take care of it.

(Letter to Jayapatāka Dāsa, October 6, 1968)

I am very anxious to know how your present condition of health is. Please let me know if you are improving. Please let me know if you are improving or if there is some disturbance still. We should always remember that our body is not for sense gratification. It is for Kṛṣṇa's service only. And to render very good sound service to Kṛṣṇa we should not neglect the upkeep of the body. We learn from an instance of Sanātana Gosvāmī. He was sometimes very much sick on account of eczema, and he was therefore sometimes bleeding. But whenever Lord Caitanya met Sanātana Gosvāmī, He used to embrace him in spite of his request for Him not to touch him. Because of this Sanātana Gosvāmī later decided to commit suicide so Lord Caitanya will not embrace him in his bloody condition. This plan was understood by Lord Caitanya, and He called Sanātana Gosvāmī and said to him, you have decided to end your body but don't you know that this body belongs to Kṛṣṇa? You have already dedicated your body so how can you decide to end it? So you must not neglect the upkeep of your body. This is the lesson we get from the Lord Caitanya and Sanātana Gosvāmī. Try to take care of your health in the best possible way.

(Letter to Rāyarāma Dāsa, February 9, 1969)

Keep your health on good condition and work very hard for Kṛṣṇa. That is our motto of life.

(Letter to Rāyarāma Dāsa, March 6, 1969)

I hope by this time your health has improved and as you are doing such important work for Kṛṣṇa, you must be careful to take proper care of your health. You are intelligent girl so conjointly with your husband,

Pradyumna, you can determine what are the best measures to be taken in this connection.

(Letter to Arundhati Dāsī, September 9, 1969)

Prabhupāda: Why everyone is coughing? What is the difficulty? Yesterday also I heard. What is the difficulty?
Devotee: I think there's a cold going around.
Prabhupāda: But you have no sufficient warm cloth, so you are affected. That you must arrange. You must take care of your health. In the *Bhagavad-gītā* it is said, *yuktāhāra*: you should take food just to maintain your health nicely. Similarly, other necessities of body must be taken care of. If you become diseased, then you can execute Kṛṣṇa consciousness? Just like Brahmānanda could not go today. So we must be careful. Better eat less than eat more. You'll not die by eating less. But you may die eating more. People die for over-eating, not for under-eating. This should be the principle. Medical science always forbids eating more than you require. Voracious eating is the cause of diabetes, and under nourishment is the cause of tuberculosis. This is the medical science. So we should not take under, neither more. Children can commit the mistake of taking more, but adults, they cannot commit. Children can digest. All day they are playing. So, anyway, we should take care of our health also. Sanātana Gosvāmī was suffering from itching very much, and Caitanya Mahāprabhu was embracing him. So these were wet itches... After itching, they became wet. So Sanātana's body was all covered with wet itches, and the moisture was sticking to the body of Caitanya Mahāprabhu. So he felt very much ashamed... And he decided, "Tomorrow I shall commit suicide instead of allowing myself to be embraced by Caitanya Mahāprabhu." So the next day Caitanya Mahāprabhu inquired, you have decided to commit suicide? So do you think this body is yours? You have already dedicated this body to Me. How you can kill it? Of course, from that day, his itches were all cured.

But this is the decision, that our body, those who are Kṛṣṇa conscious, those who are working for Kṛṣṇa, they should not think that the body belongs to them. It is already dedicated to Kṛṣṇa. So it must be kept very carefully, without any neglect. Just like you are taking care of the temple because it is Kṛṣṇa's place. We should not be over careful, but some care we should take so that we may not fall diseased.

(Lecture on Śrīmad-Bhāgavatam 1.8.37, Los Angeles, April 29, 1973)

One month, one year, whatever it takes. Disease, fire and debt are never to be neglected. Once in Bhubaneswar Gargamuni told Śrīla Prabhupāda that he had recently been very ill in Nepal. As a result he had gone down to Gopalpur on the Orissan coast for a two week break from his GBC duties to rest and recuperate. Śrīla Prabhupāda fully approved and told him that health comes first because if you aren't healthy you can't do any service.

(From Hari Śauri Dāsa)

He remained in his room throughout the morning. After breakfast he took rest and did not ring to signal he was ready for his massage until noon. He then rested again for a long time in the afternoon, and took rest early in the evening. Although he normally only sleeps three to four hours in any one day, when his body gets diseased he makes the necessary adjustments to keep it going. There doesn't seem to be any question of "good" health for Śrīla Prabhupāda; there is always something not right. But despite the hectic pace of his preaching, he is never neglectful. He deals as carefully with his body as with any other asset Kṛṣṇa has provided for his service.

(Transcendental Diary, Vol. 2, Chap. 4, May 4, 1976)

Healthy Life or Self-Preservation

In the valuable human life form, keeping the body healthy is helpful for self-realization.

Life's desires should never be directed toward sense gratification. One should desire only a healthy life, or self-preservation, since a human being is meant for inquiry about the Absolute Truth (God or Kṛṣṇa). Nothing else should be the goal of one's works.

(Śrīmad-Bhāgavatam 1.2.10)

The necessities of life for the protection and comfort of the body must not be unnecessarily increased. Human energy is spoiled in a vain search after such illusory happiness. If one is able to lie down on the floor, then why should one endeavor to get a good bedstead or soft cushion to lie on? If one can rest without any pillow and make use of the soft arms endowed by nature, there is no necessity of searching after a pillow. If we make a study of the general life of the animals, we can see that they have no intelligence for building big houses, furniture, and other household paraphernalia, and yet they maintain a healthy life by lying down on the open land. They do not know how to cook or prepare foodstuff, yet they still live healthy lives more easily than the human being. This does not mean that human civilization should revert to animal life or that the human being should live naked in the jungles without any culture, education, and sense of morality. An intelligent human cannot live the life of an animal; rather, man should try to utilize his intelligence in arts and science, poetry and philosophy. In such a way he can further the progressive march of human civilization. But here the idea given by Śrīla Śukadeva Gosvāmī is that the reserve energy of human life, which is far superior to that of animals, should simply be utilized for self-realization. Advancement of human civilization must be towards the goal of establishing our lost relationship with God, which is not possible in any form of life other than the human.

(Śrīmad-Bhāgavatam 2.2.4, purport)

Kṛṣṇa's Service Comes First

Although generally health must be given priority over other considerations, devotional service is always the first priority. Śrīla Prabhupāda's personal example is telling, for there are a number of amazing stories about how he put his service to his spiritual master and Lord *Caitanya* above any personal consideration, including his physical well-being and health.

So far as possible I am taking care of my health, but Kṛṣṇa's service must be executed even at the risk of life. A living entity gets millions of opportunities to get a type of body, but hardly he gets opportunity to serve Kṛṣṇa. The service of Kṛṣṇa must be executed at all risks, but do not worry, I am taking care of my health by the help of Gaurasundara. Hope you are well.

(Letter to Madhusūdana Dāsa, January 24, 1968)

During Śrīla Prabhupāda's massage, a Member of Parliament from

Hyderabad came to see him. The man told Prabhupāda how he had received a grant from the government of Rps. 25 lakhs (about US$250,000) to open a yoga club that will specialize in reviving ancient medicines for bodily health. Prabhupāda listened patiently and then told him candidly, "Ancient or new, it does not matter so long it does the job. By yoga you can develop the ability to walk on water, but why bother when you can pay a few paisa and cross by boat? Concentration on bodily health is simply a waste of time. Even the animals know how to look after this body." He gave the example of the mongoose, which when fighting with a snake runs off into the jungle if it gets bitten. There it finds a certain herb to eat that counteracts the venom, and then again it comes back to fight. "So even animals know how to take care of the body," he told the man. "Therefore we should take care of the soul within the body first."

(Transcendental Diary, Vol. 5, Chap. 3, November 5, 1976)

Prabhupāda felt very weak. It was on the afternoon of his appearance day, and he was sitting at his desk in the main room of his house. He lay down on his seat and put his head against one of the arm pillows. The following day he felt so weak he could not walk or stand. He had no appetite and ran a fever of 104 degrees. A local doctor arrived and examined Prabhupāda – malaria. He prescribed some medication, which Prabhupāda took once or twice and then refused. A second doctor came and prescribed different medicines. "Stop bringing these doctors," Prabhupāda said. "No doctor can cure me."

It was August, the monsoon season, and many devotees fell sick. When Śrutakīrti, who had recently returned to his post as Prabhupāda's personal servant, contracted malaria, Kulādri, who had come to Vṛndāvana to attend the temple opening, volunteered to assist. Then Kulādri got malaria. Other devotees became ill with malaria, jaundice, dysentery, and various digestive problems.

The weather was overcast, hot and humid, and thousands of varieties of insects began appearing. For several days at a time the sky would be cloudy, the temperature in the nineties. Then the sun would come out and steam everything up with almost intolerable heat. It was Vṛndāvana's most unhealthy season.

As Prabhupāda's condition worsened, the devotees became morose and even fearful for their spiritual master's life. They brought Prabhupāda's bed out where it was cooler, on the small patio outside his house. His servants would massage or fan him. Days passed and Prabhupāda didn't eat, except for a few grapes and some slices of orange. This was the way his father had died, he said-by not eating. Such remarks frightened Prabhupāda's disciples all the more, and they began visiting the *samādhis* of the Gosvāmīs to pray that Prabhupāda would be cured.

One evening Harikeśa stayed up all night near Prabhupāda's room, chanting softly a continuous *kīrtana* of Hare Kṛṣṇa. Prabhupāda liked it. "This *kīrtana*," he said, "is what actually gives us life." After that devotees took turns, so that there was always *kīrtana*.

Prabhupāda explained that his illness was due to the sins of the ISKCON leaders, eighty percent of whom were not strictly following the rules and regulations, he said. Even in Vṛndāvana some of the devotees weren't regularly rising at four A.M. Since Prabhupāda was speaking little, he had only briefly mentioned this cause of his illness. But brief as it was, it crushed his disciples. As for who was guilty, each disciple would have to say for himself. But in a mood of "Oh, God, what have we done?" all the disciples in *Vṛndavana* immediately became very attentive to the rules and regulations.

In the morning Bhāgavatam class the devotees who lectured regularly discussed the subject as explained in Śrīla Prabhupāda's books: At the time of initiation Kṛṣṇa absolves the initiate of all karmic reactions due for past sinful acts. The spiritual master, however, as the representative of Kṛṣṇa, also shares in removing the disciple's karma. Kṛṣṇa, being infinite, can never be affected by such karma, whereas the spiritual master, although completely pure, is finite. The spiritual master, therefore, partially suffers the reactions for a disciple's sins, sometimes becoming ill. Jiva Gosvāmī warns that a spiritual master should not take too many disciples, because of the danger of accepting an overload of karma. Not only does the spiritual master accept the previous karma of the disciples, but if the disciples commit sins after initiation, then for those also the spiritual master may sometimes become ill.

Prabhupāda said that his "misdeed" was accepting so many disciples, but he had no choice for spreading Kṛṣṇa consciousness. The spiritual master sometimes suffers, he said, so that the disciples may know, "Due to our sinful activities, our spiritual master is suffering," and this always had a sobering effect on any would-be offender. But now, for the first time, Prabhupāda was specifically blaming his disciples for a serious illness.

By neglecting their spiritual master's most basic instructions, they were causing him great distress. They understood that their spiritual master was no ordinary malaria victim, and they knew they had to correct their mistakes and pray to Kṛṣṇa that Prabhupāda would get better.

Prabhupāda's condition was so critical and the implications of his statements so broad that his secretary, Brahmānanda Swami, thought it best to notify the entire International Society for Kṛṣṇa Consciousness. Because Prabhupāda was pleased by the twenty-four-hour *kīrtana*, Brahmānanda Swami thought that this program might be introduced in every ISKCON temple in the world. A few telegrams were sent, and word quickly spread that every temple should hold continuous *kīrtana*, petitioning Kṛṣṇa for Prabhupāda's recovery.

It reminded some of the senior disciples of 1967, when they had stayed up all night chanting and praying for Prabhupāda's recovery from an apparent heart attack. At that time Prabhupāda had encouraged them to chant a hymn to Lord Nṛsiṁha-deva and to pray, "Our master has not finished his work. Please protect him." Due to the sincere prayers of the devotees, Prabhupāda had said, Kṛṣṇa had saved his life. Now, in 1974, there were many more devotees than in 1967, and all of them were praying for Prabhupāda's recovery; but now also, from what Prabhupāda had said, there were also more devotees to misbehave and cause him pain. That message – "Eighty percent of the leaders of my disciples are not following the rules and regulations; this is why I am suffering" – was not telegrammed. It was too heavy.

Prabhupāda had come to Vṛndāvana for a celebration, but there had been none. Now he was very sick, and his servant was carrying him in his arms to and from the bathroom. Other devotees were also massaging and serving him very sincerely. And there was always *kīrtana* for him. Meanwhile he simply depended on Kṛṣṇa and waited to get better so that he could go on with his work.

While he tolerated his condition as the mercy of Kṛṣṇa, he suddenly received word that the governor of Uttar Pradesh was coming to visit him. The governor, a Muslim named Akbar Ali Khan, was traveling in the area, and Seth Bisenchand, a friend of Prabhupāda's and the governor's, had recommended that the governor visit the temple.

Prabhupāda thought that perhaps the governor would agree to help the devotees, at least in such matters as getting government permission for steel and cement. Therefore, despite his failing health, he insisted that the devotees hold a reception in the courtyard; and he would personally go out and greet the governor. Lying on his back and speaking in a faint voice, he ordered a feast to be cooked and tables and chairs to be arranged in the courtyard.

The devotees pleaded with Prabhupāda to allow them to do everything themselves and tell the governor that Prabhupāda was very ill. "He has come," Prabhupāda said. "I have to go out and meet him."

Śrutakīrti dressed Prabhupāda in a fresh silk dhoti. Prabhupāda tried to apply the Vaiṣṇava *tilaka* to his forehead, but even that was a struggle and took more than five minutes. When they were ready to go, Prabhupāda asked his servant, "Have I put on my *tilaka*?" He seemed almost delirious from the fever and was unable to stand. Śrutakīrti and others carried him in a chair and placed him in the middle of the courtyard, where they had arranged several tables with *prasādam* and Prabhupāda's books.

Just before the governor's arrival, many policemen and soldiers arrived, roping off the area, directing traffic in front of the temple, and holding people outside until the governor arrived. Guṇārṇava had rolled a long red carpet from the edge of the property into the temple courtyard, and devotees lined both sides of the carpet, chanting with *karatālas* (cymbals) and *mṛdaṅgas* (drum). When the governor arrived, Surabhi presented him with a garland. Immediately removing the garland, the governor walked down the red carpet and into the courtyard. Prabhupāda stood.

The devotees were amazed to see Prabhupāda standing straight and shaking the governor's hand. Prabhupāda and the governor stood together for a while and then sat down. Except for the guests, everyone present knew that Prabhupāda was not capable of much exertion. They saw him shivering and trembling, yet trying to smile and be gracious with his guest. The devotees were in great anxiety, thinking that Prabhupāda's life might end at any moment, and yet they took part in the sociable pretense along with their spiritual master. The governor, on invitation, gave a speech, talking about how India's future lay in industry.

Then Prabhupāda stood to speak, leaning against his chair. His eyes were very dark, and he was barely able to focus his vision. Although he had spoken very little for almost two weeks, he now spoke for twenty minutes, while the governor listened politely. Afterward Prabhupāda sat and honored *prasādam* with the governor and his entourage of fifteen ministers. After the governor left, the devotees carried Prabhupāda back to his room, where he collapsed with a 105-degree temperature.

The political guests and military escort gone, the temple site returned to its usual quiet, and the devotees resumed their soft *kīrtana*, chanting by Prabhupāda's bedside. Amazed at Prabhupāda's strength and determination, they realized how little they themselves were actually putting forth in Kṛṣṇa consciousness.

After two full weeks Prabhupāda's fever finally broke. A great ordeal was now over. The monsoon was ending, but the same problems of temple construction persisted.

(Śrīla Prabhupāda–līlāmṛta, Chapter 44)

Two factors were making Śrīla Prabhupāda indecisive about going West. One was the worldly formalities of passport and U.S. residency card, and the other was Śrīla Prabhupāda's personal hesitancy, based on reports from the astrologer. His health was, of course, the main factor, but at times he seemed ready to disregard everything and order his servants to somehow take him to London.

(Śrīla Prabhupāda–līlāmṛta, Chapter 52)

Protect the Body

The material body is a valuable asset to use in Lord Kṛṣṇa's service; its well-being should not be neglected.

You have asked me how many hours you should work. Our life is dedicated to Kṛṣṇa and you should work for Him 24 hours. We have different varieties of service. For you, you should work on your painting as long as you think yourself fit. Don't overwork. Balance time should be spent for chanting and reading *Śrīmad-Bhāgavatam*.

(Letter to Jadurāṇī Dasi, July 8, 1967)

If you are willing to offer your medical services to my students, when it is required, that will be very nice. It is important to keep the body fit and healthy so that we will not meet the obstacle of ill health while serving Kṛṣṇa.

Ill health may hinder one's service, so we want to avoid it as much as possible.

(Letter to Dr. Currier, June 19, 1975)

The purport is that activities performed with the help of the body for the satisfaction of the Absolute Truth (*oṁ tat sat*) are never temporary, although performed by the temporary body. Indeed, such activities are everlasting. Therefore, the body should be properly cared for. Because the body is temporary, not permanent, one cannot expose the body to being devoured by a tiger or killed by an enemy. All precautions should be taken to protect the body.

(Śrīmad-Bhāgavatam 8.19.40, purport)

Pradyumna dāsa arrived this morning from Bombay. He will travel as a regular member of Śrīla Prabhupāda's party to do the Sanskrit editing on the tape transcriptions before they are sent to Los Angeles.

Pradyumna prabhu has six large boils on his hips and buttocks and cannot sit down properly. He hadn't seen a doctor so Śrīla Prabhupāda told him to get medical treatment right away. He was very concerned and not happy that Pradyumna was neglecting his health. Later in the day Pradyumna came back from the doctor's with a large bottle of the antibiotic Tetracycline which he has to take every four hours for the next ten days.

(Transcendental Diary, Vol. 2, Chap. 4, May 9, 1976)

Regulation in Habits and Simple Eating

According to Śrīmad-Bhāgavatam and Āyurvedic science, the single most important factor to keep good health is regulation, especially of eating and sleeping. If we follow the laws of nature, good health naturally follows.

Regarding your question about maintaining your body nicely, I think that if you follow our regulations of diet, sufficient sleeping and keep to the prescribed rules of cleanliness, 2 baths per day, then you will be able to keep yourself in proper health. Of course, disease will always be there at some time while there is this material body, but this we must tolerate and not be very much agitated by. Actually the Vaiṣṇava who knows that he is not this body does not therefore neglect the body, but he takes very nice care so that he may utilize this body in the service of Kṛṣṇa. Just like a man may know that he is not his car, so he does not therefore neglect his car, but he will take care of it so it will be able to render service to him. So we must take sufficient care to provide our body with its demands, but when disease or other necessary inconveniences arrive, we do not become disturbed such troubles are simply temporary manifestations.

(Letter to Balabhadra Dāsa, May 12, 1969)

Devotee: One who seeks an improvement in health or aspires . . . .
Prabhupāda: Generally this yoga practice goes on in the name of improving health. Somebody goes to reduce fat. You see? Reduce fat. Because you are rich nation, you eat more and become fatty and again pay yoga practice fees and reduce your fat. That is going on. I have seen some advertisement the other day, Reduce your fat. Why you increase your fat? The nonsense! They will not understand. That if I have to reduce it, why do I increase it? Why not be satisfied with simple foodstuff? If you eat grains and vegetables and light foodstuffs, you'll never get fatty. You see? You'll never get fatty. Reduce eating as much as possible. Don't eat at night. Practice yoga like this. If you become voracious eater, you'll be...

There are two kinds of diseases. The voracious eaters, they are attacked with diabetes and those who cannot eat sufficiently, they [will get] tuberculosis. So you cannot eat more or you cannot eat less. You just eat what you require. If you eat more then you must be diseased. And if you eat less, you must be diseased. That will be explained. *Yuktāhāra-vihārasya yogo bhavati siddhi*... You are not to starve, but don't eat more. Our program, *kṛṣṇa-prasāda*, is that you eat *kṛṣṇa-prasāda*.

Eating is required; you have to keep your body fit for any practice. So eating is required. But don't eat more. Don't eat less also. We don't say that you eat less. If you can eat ten pounds, eat. But if you cannot eat ten pounds, out of avarice, out of greediness you eat pounds, then you will suffer. You see?

(Lecture on Bhagavad-gītā 6.13–15, Los Angeles, February 16, 1969)

In the kali-Yuga, the duration of life is shortened not so much because of insufficient food but because of irregular habits. By keeping regular habits and eating simple food, any man can maintain his health. Overeating, over-sense gratification, over dependence on another's mercy, and artificial standards of living sap the very vitality of human energy. Therefore the duration of life is shortened.

(Śrīmad-Bhāgavatam 1.1.10, purport)

Prabhupāda's Daily Schedule

It is hard to say when Prabhupāda's day begins and when it ends, because he never seems to conclude his activities in the way we do. He only rests for a few hours each day, and even that is intermittent.
Śrīla Prabhupāda maintains a remarkably regulated daily routine. While here in Vṛndāvana his schedule is:

6:00 a.m. -- Wash, brush teeth, and take Āyurvedic medicine.
6:30 - 7:30 a.m. -- Morning walk.
7:30 - 8:30 a.m. -- Greet the Deities, *guru-pūjä*, then *Śrīmad-Bhāgavatam* lecture from the Seventh Canto.
9:00 - 9:30 a.m. -- Breakfast of fruits and *chīra* (fried rice sometimes with nuts).
9:45 - 11:15 a.m. -- Rest on roof for an hour and then meet people (usually by appointment).
11:15 - 1:15 p.m. -- Massage with oil.
1:15 - 1:45 p.m. -- Bathe.
1:45 - 2:30 p.m. -- Lunch prasādam.
2:30 - 3:00 p.m. -- Sit in room or chant japa (soft recitation of God's names on beads).
3:00 - 4:00 p.m. -- Rest.
4:00 - 5:00 p.m. -- Meet with specific people or devotees, or chant.
5:00 - 6:30 p.m. -- Give public *darśana* (interview).
6:30 - 9:30 p.m. -- Meet public or senior devotees, GBC business or just chat.
9:30 p.m. -- Take hot milk, massage and rest.
12:00 - 1:00 a.m. -- Rise and translate.
5:00 a.m. -- Light rest or japa.
Śrīla Prabhupāda's typical routine goes something like today.

After his all-night translation work he stopped at *maṅgala-ārātrika* (ceremony to worship the Deity early in the morning) time and lay back against the bolsters with his feet up. He slept lightly for a short time.

At six o'clock he went into the bathroom to wash, brush his teeth, and freshen up. He came back and sat for a few minutes as he put on *tilaka*. When that was completed, he took a reddish Āyurvedic medicinal pellet called Yogendra-rasa. After I had crushed it with a large, roasted cardamom seed and then mixed it with honey in a small oval mortar, he added a little water. He drank the mixture straight from the mortar, scraping up the residue with the pestle, which he then deposited on his tongue with an elegant twist of his fingers.

Then Prabhupāda prepared to leave for his morning walk. Getting up from his desk he stood patiently as I helped him on first with his *uttarīya* (the saffron top-piece traditionally worn by all *sannyāsīs*) then with his heavy saffron-colored coat and his woolen hat. I finally hung his bead bag around his neck. All the while he conversed with Haṅsadūta, Akṣayānanda Swami, and Gopāla Kṛṣṇa.

As he walked toward the door, I rushed ahead to place his cane directly into his hand. I then positioned his shoes so that he could step into them and out of his slippers in one easy movement, all while I was holding the door open. It is somewhat of an art to manage all this without delaying or interrupting Prabhupāda's steady progress out.

(Transcendental Diary, Vol. 1, Chap. 2, Dec. 5, 1975)

Gurukula Schedule

When they discussed *prasādam* times, Prabhupāda told them that the period from rising at 3:30 to breakfast at 9:30 was too long for the children to go without eating. They should be given *maṅgala-ārati* sweets immediately after the *ārati*. And when informed that they had a second bath at 12:30, he said that they should not bathe for at least four hours after eating, but he was happy with their taking lunch at about one o'clock and then resting for an hour after before attending their afternoon Sanskrit class

(Transcendental Diary, Vol. 5, Chap. 3, November 5, 1976)

Life not so long ago in India, he said, was very simple and pleasant. "In India they don't require even cottage. One *katiya* [wooden cot] is sufficient.

Keeping in one place and lay down. Eight months, at least six months, it is very nice. At night – even in daytime it is very hot – at night it is cool. So you have got very good sleep, soothing, then you become refreshed in the morning. If you have got good sleep at night, then you become refreshed; your health is regained. Hmm? Take morning *snāna* (bath) and *chapati* (unleavened flat bread). During very hot season they don't take even *chapati*. They take some fruits, guava, and melon, yes. During hot season you get watermelon, this other melon, honeydew melon – oh very nice! In the upcountries still in the village during daytime they don't eat. During daytime they take some fruits, and at night when it is cool, the cool refreshing air, they make some *chapati*. Because in daytime it is so hot, it is embarrassing to cook and to digest also. Better take fruit, this melon, and at night they take three or four *chapati*, and good sleep. Very happy life it was, all over India. There was no question of poverty. People did not know what is poverty, and now it is poverty. They do not get even sufficient food."

"Industrialization," I observed.

Prabhupāda nodded. "*ugra-karma*. I don't like industrialism."

(Transcendental Diary, Volume 5, Chap. 3, November 3, 1976)

Kiśorī Dāsī and other ladies prepared Prabhupāda's breakfast. It consisted of various cut fruits: seedless grapes, guava, banana, orange, pomegranate, and whatever else was freshly available at the market. With this he had a small bowl of fried *chīra*, another of fried cashew nuts, and a small piece of *sandeśa* milk sweet. One item is vital to Prabhupāda's breakfast: ginger soaked in lemon juice. He won't start breakfast without it, as it stimulates his digestion.

Śrīla Prabhupāda ate little and very slowly, as an act of devotion: *prasāda-sevā*, service, rather than indulging the tongue. When he finished, I cleared his plate and wiped the table as he sat and cleaned his teeth. It surprised me to see that his teeth moved apart when he inserted the wooden pick, but Prabhupāda just laughed about it.

When he finished he held out his open palm for me to tip a little *bhāskar lavan*, an Āyurvedic digestive powder, into it. Tilting his head back, he dropped in the powder. Then still maintaining the pose, he poured in some water from the tumbler without touching it to his lips. After washing his mouth and hands in the bathroom he returned to his *darśana* room.

(Transcendental Diary, Vol. 1, Chap.2, December 5, 1975)

Speaking from *Śrīmad*-Bhāgavatam 6.1.12 in his class, Śrīla Prabhupāda continued to stress the need for culture. His lecture was short but direct and very much to the point. He made it clear what he meant by culture. "The Vedic civilization means everything under rules and regulation. That is Vedic civilization. Animal cannot be brought under rules and regulations. That is not possible. That is the specialty of the human society, that the more one society follows rules and regulations, he is to be considered civilized."

He gave the English translation of the verse, which unequivocally describes the need for regulated life. "My dear King, if a diseased person eats the pure, uncontaminated food prescribed by a physician, he is gradually cured, and the infection of disease can no longer touch him. Similarly, if one follows the regulative principles of knowledge, he gradually progresses toward liberation from material contamination."

Prabhupāda repeatedly stressed this point – unless we follow the rules and regulations, then there is no possibility of curing our material disease. Thus he also indicated the need for the establishment of a society like his ISKCON.

"The law is meant for the human being. If the human being does not follow rules and regulative principle, law, then he's animal. So civilized means to raise oneself from the animal status of life to the human status life. That means rules and regulations. That is compulsory, that is human… Real civilization is how to go back to home, back to Godhead, but materialistic persons do not know this. Therefore there must be organization, institution, to teach the human society how to go back to home, back to Godhead."

(Transcendental Diary, Vol. 2, Chap. 4, May 13, 1976)

Teach Them Not to Fall Sick

Knowledge about how to remain healthy and avoid sickness counteracts the sinful activities caused by ignorance in modern society.

Prabhupāda: Patient is always rascal fool. You cannot expect him to be intelligent. He must agree to the physician's directions. That is intelligence.

He must know that he's diseased; he must follow the instruction of the physician. That much will help him. Unless one is rascal, he does not fall sick. As soon as you violate the hygienic principles, you become sick. All commit sinful activities on account of ignorance. So therefore the best advancement of civilization is not to open hospitals, but to give them a lesson that they may not fall sick and go to hospitals. That is real...But they do not know. They keep the mass of people in ignorance, they fall sick and they come to hospital and number of hospitals increase, they think it is advancement. This is their idea.

(Conversation, New Vrindaban, June 23, 1976)

Don't Misuse the Body, Use It for Freedom

Youthful energy is an asset that's properly engaged when used to perform devotional service and advance in Kṛṣṇa consciousness.

Therefore, while in material existence [*bhavam āśritaḥ*], a person fully competent to distinguish wrong from right must endeavor to achieve the highest goal of life as long as the body is stout and strong and is not embarrassed by dwindling.

(Śrīmad-Bhāgavatam 7.6.5)

The highest goal of life can be achieved as long as one's body is stout and strong. We should therefore live in such a way that we keep ourselves always healthy and strong in mind and intelligence so that we can distinguish the goal of life from a life full of problems. A thoughtful man must act in this way, learning to distinguish right from wrong, and thus attain the goal of life.

(Śrīmad-Bhāgavatam 7.6.5, purport)

Even if for the sake of argument the material world is accepted as untruth, the living entity entangled in the illusory energy cannot come out of it without the help of the body. Without the help of the body, one cannot follow a system of religion, nor can one speculate on philosophical perfection. Therefore, the flower and fruit (*puṣpa-phalam*) have to be obtained as a result of the body. Without the help of the body, that fruit cannot be gained.

[Yukta-vairāga is the spiritual detachment that comes from using things not for one's own sense gratification, but for the pleasure of the Supreme Lord.]

The Vaiṣṇava philosophy therefore recommends *yukta-vairāgya*. It is not that all attention should be diverted for the maintenance of the body, but at the same time one's bodily maintenance should not be neglected.

As long as the body exists one can thoroughly study the Vedic instructions, and thus at the end of life one can achieve perfection. This is explained in *Bhagavad-gītā* [Bg. 8.6]: *yaṁ yaṁ vāpi smaran bhāvaṁ tyajaty ante kalevaram*. Everything is examined at the time of death. Therefore, although the body is temporary, not eternal, one can take from it the best service and make one's life perfect.

(Śrīmad-Bhāgavatam 8.19.39, purport)

In this respect, the young Prahlāda Mahārāja's instructions are particularly important for us. This morning's Śrīmad-Bhāgavatam verse (7.6.5) spoke precisely on this theme of taking full advantage of one's youth for spiritual attainment. The translation was, "For this reason, a person who is fully competent to distinguish wrong and right while keeping himself in material existence, *bhāvam āśritāḥ*, must endeavor for achieving the highest goal of life so long the body is stout and strong and is not embarrassed by the dwindling condition of life." Śrīla Prabhupāda commented, "Nobody wants to become old man, especially in this winter season. It is very difficult for old men. So, you have to accept *jarā* (old age) and *vyādhi* (disease). Nobody can escape disease. When I am diseased there is a great struggle how to cure myself, go to the doctor, take good medicine, and so on. But we cannot check the diseased condition. Similarly we cannot check our old age, cannot check our birth, death. Therefore here it is said, *kuśalāḥ*. *Kuśalāḥ* means if you actually want benefit, because this kind of struggling has not given you any benefit, *tato yateta*, then you should endeavor for this. What is that? *Kṣemāya*, for your ultimate benefit.And how long? *Śarīraṁ puruṣaṁ yāvan na vipadyeta puṣkalam*. So long you are stout and strong you should try how to become free from this bondage of birth, death, old age, and disease. Not that you keep this business set aside, 'When we shall get old then we shall chant Hare Kṛṣṇa and become Kṛṣṇa conscious.'

(Transcendental Diary, Vol. 1, Chap.2, December 7, 1975)

Prabhupāda unfolded upon us the deep realizations he has gained from a lifetime's devotional practice and ten years of constant global travel, witnessing the activities of every class of man in almost every culture of the world. He stressed the need for us to capitalize on the good facility we have with our still-youthful bodies. "So long we are stout and strong and we can work very nicely, the health is quite all right, take advantage of it. It is not Kṛṣṇa consciousness movement is for the lazy fellow. No. It is meant for the strong man. Strong in body, strong in mind, strong in determination, everything strong. Strong in brain, it is meant for them because we have to execute the highest goal of life."

(Transcendental Diary, Vol. 2, Chap.7, June 21, 1976)

Pure Mind and Hygienic in Body

A mahājana's instruction on purity and health.

Bhīṣmadeva advised for all human beings nine qualifications: (1) not to become angry, (2) not to lie, (3) distribute wealth, (4) to forgive, (5) to beget children only by one's legitimate wife, (6) to be pure in mind and hygienic in body, (7) not to be inimical toward anyone, (8) to be simple, and (9) to support servants or subordinates. One cannot be called a civilized person without acquiring the above-mentioned preliminary qualities.

(Śrīmad-Bhāgavatam 1.9.26, purport)

Best Use of a Bad Bargain

The aim of human life is not to enjoy perverted sense enjoyment but to cure the material disease by developing spiritual knowledge. To do this, you need the help of the body and the mind. Therefore, if we are to reach our goal, maintenance of the body and mind is required.

We have to plan our activities in such a way that we become stronger, not weaker. Physically I am becoming weak, so you boys become stronger.
(Letter to Tamāla Kṛṣṇa Mahārāja, August 13, 1974)

The principal rules and regulations in the Hare Kṛṣṇa Movement is not to eat meat, fish or eggs; not to engage in sex outside of marriage with the purpose of producing children to raise in God consciousness, no gambling, no intoxication. Not following these principles is unhealthy for the body, mind and soul. "Chanting 16 rounds daily" refers to chanting the names of God on beads, which are similar to a rosary, a certain number of times around a day.

Regarding Bhūmātā devī dāsī's affliction, she should simply take the proper treatment. Make the best out of a bad bargain. This material body is a bad bargain because it is always miserable. So, to make the best out of this bad bargain means to render devotional service in any circumstance. The dust from the lotus feet of the spiritual master is never to be used for material benefit. That is a great misconception. The best thing is that the girl tries her best to chant 16 rounds daily and to follow all the rules and regulations even if she is afflicted with something, and in this way she will fully understand the mercy of Kṛṣṇa and the spiritual master.
(Letter to Kṛṣṇanandiṇī Dāsī, April 8, 1975)

There are many examples in history of persons who have been very much disabled physically, but still have executed Kṛṣṇa consciousness. Still, up to date in places like Vṛndāvana, India, there are many persons who are blind, crippled, lame, deformed, etc., but they are determined to practice Kṛṣṇa consciousness to their best ability. So, you should also do like that. Simply be determined to practice the process of Bhakti-yoga (The science of devotion to the Supreme Lord) with whatever abilities you may have. If you are really sincere, then Kṛṣṇa will give you help. If you require any medical help, you can take as much as is needed.
(Letter to Kṛṣṇa Vilāsinī Dāsī, June 3, 1975)

As long as the body will be there, there will only he pain. Pleasure is only a misconception. Do not be sorry if you are in an 'unfortunate' situation. It can also be fortunate if you take advantage by becoming serious to become

Kṛṣṇa conscious. Follow the regulative principles, chant sixteen rounds and as far as possible render service and study my books. Success is sure.

(Letter to Kṛṣṇa Vilāsinī Dāsī, October 25, 1976)

The Vedas enjoin that the factual result of the tree of the body is the good fruits and flowers derived from it. But if the bodily tree does not exist, there is no possibility of factual fruits and flowers. Even if the body is based on untruth, there cannot be factual fruits and flowers without the help of the bodily tree.

PURPORT

This *Śloka* explains that in relation to the material body even the factual truth cannot exist without a touch of untruth. The Māyāvādīs say, *brahmā satyaṁ jagan mithyā*: "The spirit soul is truth, and the external energy is untruth." The Vaiṣṇava philosophers, however, do not agree with the Māyāvāda philosophy. Even if for the sake of argument the material world is accepted as untruth, the living entity entangled in the illusory energy cannot come out of it without the help of the body. Without the help of the body, one cannot follow a system of religion, nor can one speculate on philosophical perfection. Therefore, the flower and fruit (*puṣpa-phalam*) have to be obtained as a result of the body. Without the help of the body, that fruit cannot be gained. The Vaiṣṇava philosophy therefore recommends *yukta-vairāgya*. It is not that all attention should be diverted for the maintenance of the body, but at the same time one's bodily maintenance should not be neglected. As long as the body exists one can thoroughly study the Vedic instructions, and thus at the end of life one can achieve perfection. This is explained in *Bhagavad-gītā* [Bg. 8.6]: *yaṁ yaṁ vāpi smaran bhāvaṁ tyajaty ante kalevaram*. Everything is examined at the time of death. Therefore, although the body is temporary, not eternal, one can take from it the best service and make one's life perfect.

*(Śrīmad-*Bhāgavatam *8.19.39, and purport)*

Real sense enjoyment is possible only when the disease of materialism is removed. In our pure spiritual form, free from all material contamination, real enjoyment of the senses is possible. A patient must regain his health before he can truly enjoy sense pleasure again. Thus the aim of human life should not be to enjoy perverted sense enjoyment but to cure the material disease. Aggravation of the material disease is no sign of knowledge, but a sign of *avidyā*, ignorance. For good health, a person should not increase his fever from 105 degrees to 107 degrees but should reduce his temperature to the normal 98.6. That should be the aim of human life. The modern trend of material civilization is to increase the temperature of the feverish material condition, which has reached the point of 107 degrees in the form of atomic energy. Meanwhile, the foolish politicians are crying that at any moment the world may go to hell. That is the result of the advancement of material knowledge and the neglect of the most important part of life, the culture of spiritual knowledge. . . . we must not follow this dangerous path leading to death. On the contrary, we must develop the culture of spiritual knowledge so that we may become completely free from the cruel hands of death.

This does not mean that all activities for the maintenance of the body should be stopped. There is no question of stopping activities, just as there is no question of wiping out one's temperature altogether when trying to recover from a disease. To make the best use of a bad bargain is the appropriate expression. The culture of spiritual knowledge necessitates the help of the body and mind; therefore maintenance of the body and mind is required if we are to reach our goal. The normal temperature should be maintained at 98.6 degrees, and the great sages and saints of India have attempted to do this by a balanced program of spiritual and material knowledge. They never allow the misuse of human intelligence for diseased sense gratification.

(Śrī Īśopaniṣad, Mantra 11, purport)

Dr. Wolfe: Can one say that the soul and life are identical?
Prabhupāda: Yes. Identical. Life is the symptom of the soul. Because the soul is there, therefore life is there. And as soon the soul is not there, there is no more life. There is sun in the sky, and the light is there, sunshine. When the sun is set, there is no more light; it is dark.
Dr. Pore: Is the body, then, to be resisted? Is the body to be disciplined, to be resisted, to be ignored? Is that what you're suggesting?
Prabhupāda: Ignored?
Dr. Pore: How do you treat the body?

Prabhupāda: Make the best use of a bad bargain [laughter]. It is a bad bargain. But we have to utilize it.
Dr. Pore: When you say, then, that everything is a part of God, you make an exception of the body, the body is not.
Prabhupāda: No, why? Body is also part. That I explained.
Dr. Judah: *Māyā-Śakti* (illusionary material energy).
Prabhupāda: Yes, it is another energy.
Dr. Pore: Oh, I see.
Dr. Judah: The inferior energy of Kṛṣṇa.
Prabhupāda: Everything is God's energy, so the body is also God's energy. So best use of the body is God's energy should be utilized for God. Then the body is spiritualized. The body is also God's energy, and when it is utilized in God's service, it is no longer a bad bargain, it is a good bargain.
(Conversation, June 24, 1975)

At the same time, warning signs of His Divine Grace's (title given to a spiritual master as a pure representative of God) deteriorating health grew stronger. He suffered attacks of toothache, high blood pressure, heart palpitations, kidney disease and flu all with stoic indifference, and relentlessly pushed himself on despite his weakening bodily condition. It was both distressing and impressive for his servants – distressing because there was very little we could do to relieve him, and impressive because we saw his great and selfless determination to use his body to the last breath in the service of Lord Kṛṣṇa and humanity at large.
(Transcendental Diary, Vol. 3, Preface)

Old House

When the body gets old, don't expect good health.

Regarding my health, I am glad to inform you that it is in better condition than that of last year when I returned from India. I am feeling no more headaches nor any severe buzzing sound—but still some buzzing is going on. After all, it is a broken house and I cannot expect all the comforts of a newly built house in an old broken residence.
(Letter to Brahmānanda, December 19, 1968)

Yes, the same things are going on. I am trying to change diets and sometimes fasting. But after all, it is old body, so dizziness is not unnatural.

(Letter to Himavatī Dāsī, April 1, 1970)

For the time being I am keeping my health fairly well. Certainly I was sick when I left Calcutta for London, but I improved my health there. So after all, this is an old body. I am 78 years, and still by the grace of Kṛṣṇa it is going on. So I am very much thankful for your enquiry about my health.

(Letter to Dinesh Candra Sarkar, November 9, 1973)

Since we arrived Prabhupāda has been resting until late in the morning, after 7 a.m. He has not taken a full morning walk since leaving New York. This morning he ate very little for breakfast. He also told us to make all endeavor necessary to prevent him from catching cold. He said that, "With an old body, it means thin blood, and this turns to mucus. And when there is too much mucus it blocks the heart, and this is very dangerous." He has spent the last couple of days sitting quietly in his room, but at least he is once again having his massage in the sunshine and taking a full bath.

(Transcendental Diary, Vol. 3, Chap. 5, July 31, 1976)

Prabhupāda's health is not very good. He has been suffering from high blood pressure for several days, and today he has toothache. Indeed, he seems to be suffering a general decline in health and strength. At this time last year he was striding strongly down the road every morning for at least one hour and seemed quite full of vigor. Now he rarely takes such walks.

Last December he once rose from his desk, radiant with youthful energy, and declared, "I am not an old man. I will never grow old!" Now, just the other day, as I followed him up the staircase to go up onto the roof, I watched as he strained to get to the top, pushing himself up the last few steps with his cane. He paused for a moment to rest and, half-turning to me, said with a smile, "Now I am old."

(Transcendental Diary, Vol. 4, Chap. 5, September 11, 1976)

One morning Śrīla Prabhupāda asked for orange juice, but there were no oranges in the kitchen. Gopīnātha ran to get them, but when he returned, Śrīla Prabhupāda was ringing his bell. Gopīnātha rushed in and told him, "I am just coming. It takes time to make the juice." After a few minutes, when the juice did not come, Śrīla Prabhupāda began repeatedly ringing his bell. As Gopīnātha at last entered with the juice, Prabhupāda spoke out angrily, "I am sick with no appetite, and when I have a little hunger, then you take hours!" He said he didn't want the juice, but Gopīnātha put it on the table anyway.

Śrīla Prabhupāda picked the glass up and drank. "You are serving me so nicely," he said quietly. "I am always chastising you. When one gets old, he becomes short-tempered." Gopīnātha had not felt bad about the reprimand, but on these humble words from Śrīla Prabhupāda he felt terrible. Gopīnātha became so emotional that he could hardly speak. Yet he managed, in a choked voice, to say, "Please, Śrīla Prabhupāda, don't speak like that. I make mistakes, and if you don't correct them, then who will?"

(Śrīla Prabhupāda-līlāmṛta, Chap 51)

Not Too Cold

When the body gets old, it's sometimes more difficult to tolerate the cold.

I am very much anxious to go to Europe to visit London, Germany and other places as soon as there is opportunity. The only problem is it should not be too cold for me, an old man. So you let me know the maximum temperature at the present moment, or if in the month of March the climate will be all right. I can tolerate very nicely temperatures of 50–60 degrees.

(Letter to Kṛṣṇa Dāsa, February 13, 1969)

Tolerance

Bodily miseries will come and go. We have to tolerate them and try to advance in Kṛṣṇa consciousness.

So long we have got this material body, the miseries will be coming and going, simply we have to tolerate them and try to make advancement in Kṛṣṇa consciousness as best as we can.

(Letter to Pradyumna Dāsa, March 23, 1968)

I am in due receipt of your very nice letter and I am both happy and unhappy on reading it. I am happy to hear from you, but I am unhappy because I hear that for the last 3 months you are not keeping your good health. I do not know why you should reduce in your health, but after all, this body is external—we should not be very much disturbed with it. It is advised in the *Bhagavad-gītā* that this bodily happiness and unhappiness are temporary, like seasonal changes, so we are not very much disturbed even in severe cold or scorching heat, we have to execute our daily duties, we may not be very much disturbed with our bodily pains. But because we are long associated with this material body, sometimes we are afflicted, but by higher knowledge we have to tolerate the pains, wisely thinking that these bodily pains are not mine.

(Letter to Yamunā Dāsī, March 13, 1969)

So far your health is concerned, so far the body is there the question of health and unhealth will always be there. Sometimes there will be complaints, and sometimes not. In the *Gita* (*Bhagavad-gītā*) Kṛṣṇa says these things come and go like the seasonal changes. So we have to tolerate. Caitanya Mahāprabhu advises: *tṛṇād api sunīcena taror api sahiṣṇunā.* We must be tolerant like the tree and humble like the blade of grass. Such persons can chant the Hare Kṛṣṇa mantra and preach. In Bombay we are undergoing so many tribulations. What can be done?

(Letter to Subāla Dāsa Swami, November 25, 1974)

The best thing for your wife is to try and tolerate the pains and to execute her devotional service to the best of her capacity. If this is difficult, then she should try to get the proper treatment for her problem. And in this case, you may consult with Jagadīśa dāsa for advice. Under any circumstances, she should follow all the rules and regulations and chant at least sixteen good rounds daily.

(Letter to Jitasvāra Dāsa, April 17, 1975)

The girl who has got health problems must learn to be tolerant. As long as the material body will be there, there will only be pain. Pleasure is a misconception.

(Letter to Bala Kṛṣṇa Dāsa, October 23, 1976)

Temple of Disease

Expect the body to give problems and chant Hare Kṛṣṇa.

You don't worry about my health. I am quite fit now and in New Vṛndāvana I am walking on the hills daily. In Boston for 3 or 4 days I had some acute backache pain but by the grace of Kṛṣṇa it was made all right very soon. This body is called the temple of diseases. So long as there is no disease it is wonderful, but when there is disease it is not wonderful. So this is the temple of disease. Of course, you are all very kind upon me, whenever I am slightly indisposed you become concerned, and I thank you very much for such anxiety. But so far as I am concerned, I always wish only to expedite my mission of life to spread Kṛṣṇa consciousness in the Western part of the world. I am still firmly convinced that if I can establish this movement through the help of all the boys and girls who have now joined with me, then it will be a great advancement.

I am old man, and there has already been warning, but before I leave this body, I wish to see some of you very strong in Kṛṣṇa consciousness understanding. I am very glad and proud also that you six boys and girls, although you have not been able to establish a nice center in London, still you have done your best. And the news has reached far away in India that my disciples are doing very nice work in Kṛṣṇa consciousness. So that is my pride.

(Letter to Mukunda Dāsa, May 27, 1969)

Prabhupāda asked about Kīrtanānanda's health, and Mahārāja explained that he has been suffering due to some paralysis in his left arm. Prabhupāda didn't register much concern, telling him not to worry. He said we should expect the body to give us trouble. We must simply take shelter of the holy names of the Lord.

(Transcendental Diary, Vol. 1, Chap. 4, December 18, 1975)

janma-mṛtyu-jarā-vyādhi **(birth, death, old age and disease) are the most important problems of life to solve. Unfortunately, people are not educated in the solution to these problems, namely to revive our eternal relationship with the Supreme Lord and thus**

become aware of our spiritual identity beyond our present gross and subtle material covering.

A few pieces of mail have been forwarded here, and Prabhupāda answered them as he took his massage. An old associate of Prabhupāda's, Dinesh Candra Sarkar, wrote from Calcutta, enquiring about Prabhupāda's health and activities since he saw him in Māyāpur last March. He related how he had been bed-ridden with bronchitis and pneumonia for two months and now is so weak that he is unable to travel to either Māyāpur or the Calcutta temple. He begged for Śrīla Prabhupāda's blessings and some news of when he will return to Māyāpur.

Prabhupāda sympathized with him over his poor health, briefly recounting his own health troubles of the cold he caught in New York. "So I am sorry to learn that you are not well. Pray to Kṛṣṇa and chant Hare Kṛṣṇa. The body is a temple of disease, *janma-mṛtyu-jarā-vyādhi*. Disease is our inevitable companion. We still have to execute our duty of Kṛṣṇa consciousness as far as possible and Kṛṣṇa will help us."

(Transcendental Diary, Vol. 4, Chap. 4, August 26, 1976)

Woman's Health and Having Children

Before trying to have children, a woman should be in good health.

I am sorry to hear of your wife's poor health. You have tried so many treatments, pills and better climates and visits to doctors, but there is no improvement. I think you can admit her to the hospital on a longer term basis for recouping her health. You should not expect to have children until she is in good health.

(Letter to Muralīdhara Dāsa, June 9, 1974)

Don't Leave Remnants of Food

Devotees do not leave food remnants.

Śrī Caitanya Mahāprabhu said, "I will not be able to eat so much food, and it is not the duty of a sannyāsī to leave remnants."

(Caitanya-caritāmṛta, Madhya-līlā 3.74*)*

According to Śrīmad-Bhāgavatam (11.18.19):

bahir jalāśayaṁ gatvā tatopaspṛśya vāg-yataḥ
vibhajya pāvitaṁ śeṣaṁ bhuñjītāśeṣam āhṛtam

"Whatever edibles a sannyāsī gets from a householder's house he should take outside near some lake or river, and after offering the food to Viṣṇu, Brahmā and the sun (three divisions), he should eat the entire offering and not leave anything for others to eat."

(Caitanya-caritamrta, Madhya-līlā 3.74, purport)

When preparing Śrīla Prabhupāda's lunch yesterday, I discovered that the only salt available came in large crystalline lumps that had to be broken and crushed. Because this was somewhat troublesome, I spent half an hour making enough for the following few days, and put the small stone bowl containing the salt on Prabhupāda's *choṇki* (small table to eat on). I assumed that Prabhupāda would take as much as he wanted from the stock and leave the rest for future use.

During breakfast, however, Prabhupāda dipped pieces of fruit directly into the bowl rather than taking some salt from it onto his plate and leaving the rest. When I cleaned up afterwards I left the salt bowl on the table, thinking it would be all right to use it for other meals.

Though conversing with the other devotees, Śrīla Prabhupāda, as observant as ever, noticed what I did and immediately rebuked me. Calling me a *yavana* he complained about our Western eating habit of saving remnants of food. "There is no taste, no vitamin, and still they eat."

Harikeśa asked if it would be all right if I kept the salt in the pot, and then put some on the plate when Prabhupāda took his *prasādam*.

"I do not know whether it is all right, but it is not all right that you eat and keep it. This is not all right."

Yaśodānandana explained, "He keeps the salt in a separate bowl. When you require it, he will give you only as much as you require."

Prabhupāda said, "Yes, that is nice."

"That's why the bowl is there," I explained. "That's what I intended to do, but I have to keep it away from the table."

Prabhupāda said, "The principle should be that you should not leave remnants of food. As soon as it is used, it should not be used more. Otherwise it is not possible to give up. *Paraṁ dṛṣṭvā nivartate.* "I am eating something not very superior, but if I get the chance of eating something superior then I give up this inferior."

(Transcendental Diary, Vol. 1, Chap. 7, January 4, 1976)

Duties in Relation to the Body and Mind

Anything done to please Lord Kṛṣṇa, even in relationship to the body and the mind, is devotional service.

Your cooking business is not stopped. Simply the mode of thinking has to be changed. That's all. A small technique that I am earning for God. I am eating also for God. How is that eating you are...? Now, because my body is dedicated to the service of the Lord, if I don´t eat sufficiently to keep my body work? So your eating is also God consciousness. Your sleeping is also consciousness. So that is the way. We have to mold our life's activities. Now, when I think that I have to keep this body fit for working for God, so then that is not, I mean to...That is not bodily conception of life. Just like when you think that My car has to be kept very nicely so that I can take some service of the car. Similarly, if you think that "This body is required for acting, for working on behalf of the Supreme Lord; therefore I must keep the body fit to work," so that is not your identification with the body for sense gratification and therefore I make my body stout and strong to enjoy sense enjoyment, that is the cause of my bondage.

(Lecture on Bhagavad-gītā 2.48–49, New York, April 1, 1966)

Bhaktivinoda Ṭhākura warns us in this connection that we should not mistakenly think that the idea of giving up everything implies the renunciation of duties necessary in relation to the body and mind. Even such duties are not sense gratification if they are undertaken in a spirit of service to Kṛṣṇa.

(Caitanya-caritamrta, Ādi-līlā 4.170, purport)

Now, whatever affection we see the *gopīs* show for their own bodies, know it for certain to be only for the sake of Lord Kṛṣṇa.

[The *gopīs* think:] "I have offered this body to Lord Kṛṣṇa. He is its owner, and it brings Him enjoyment. Kṛṣṇa finds joy in seeing and touching this body." It is for this reason that they cleanse and decorate their bodies.

"O Arjuna, there are no greater receptacles of deep love for Me than the *gopīs*, who cleanse and decorate their bodies because they consider them Mine."

(Caitanya-caritamrta, Ādi-lilā 4.181–184)

Don't Bother Very Much with the Body

The body will be vanquished today or tomorrow, but we have to continue our devotional service in Kṛṣṇa consciousness.

Regarding my backache, the 10% balance appears to be out of my body, but after all, the material body can be infected at any time, so we should not bother very much about it. We must simply go on with our activities in Kṛṣṇa consciousness.

(Letter to Tamāl Kṛṣṇa Dāsa, May 6, 1969)

This body is today or tomorrow finished. We should not be very much bothered about the body. Trees also live for thousands of years but that does not mean a successful life. A successful life is one of Kṛṣṇa consciousness. By the grace of Kṛṣṇa from the very beginning you are a devotee and that is the real profit of your life.

I thank you for your check, but I would prefer that you may require the money for your treatment. So if you like I can return it. But I hear that you have some income. I pray to Kṛṣṇa for your more advanced Kṛṣṇa conscious life. About a sadhu (saintly person) it is said: *jīva vā maro sādhur*, a sadhu may live or die, it doesn't matter. While living he is engaged in Kṛṣṇa conscious business and when dying he goes back home back to Godhead. Hoping this finds you improving in your health.

(Letter to Jayānanda Dāsa, February 26, 1977)

Chapter 2
Health and Sickness in Spiritual Life

Everything Depends on Kṛṣṇa

Lord Kṛṣṇa is the master of everything, including our health and disease.

So far my health is concerned, on the whole it is nice, but sometimes I feel not so good. Everything depends on Kṛṣṇa, as He desires it will happen.
(Letter to Brahmānanda Dāsa, July 11, 1967)

In the meantime try to recoup your health, depending on Kṛṣṇa, because after all He is the ultimate Master of all situations. It is not the doctor, or the medicine, or the place, but it is ultimately Kṛṣṇa Who is the Master to do everything. With this viewpoint we shall go forward.
(Letter to Rāyarāma Dāsa, March 20, 1969)

I am happy to hear you are very much liking living in New Vṛndāvana, and that you are anxiously awaiting receipt of your first cow. I am also very much concerned about your health. I have written Hayagrīva in this connection. But I do not know what could be the cause of this illness. Please let me know what are the reports given by the doctor. But it is good that you are keeping even greater amount of faith in Kṛṣṇa, and are chanting 35 rounds daily. Keep up this good attitude and surely you will be saved from all dangers.
(Letter to Śyāmā Dāsī, March 24, 1969)

Grossly materialistic persons think that economic development is of foremost importance because they are under the impression that a living entity exists only by eating. Such grossly materialistic persons forget that although we may eat as much as we like, if the food is not digested it produces the troubles of indigestion and acidity. Therefore, eating is not in itself the cause of the vital energy of life. For digestion of eatables we have to take shelter of another, superior energy, which is mentioned in the *Bhagavad-gītā* as *vaiśvānara*. Lord Kṛṣṇa says in the *Bhagavad-gītā* that He helps the digestion in the form of *vaiśvānara*. The Supreme Personality of Godhead is all-pervasive; therefore, His presence in the stomach as *vaiśvānara* is not extraordinary.

(Kṛṣṇa The Supreme Personality of Godhead, Chapter 87)

Work on the Spiritual Platform

Even if there is some disease, we must maintain ourselves on the spiritual platform.

Physically and mentally we may be disturbed sometimes, but we have to stand erect on the spiritual platform. I may inform you in this connection that I am at the present moment physically unfit; I am having always a buzzing sound in my brain. I cannot sleep soundly at night, but still I am working because I try to be on the spiritual platform. I hope you shall try to understand me right, and do the needful. Hope you are well.

(Letter to Yamunā Devī Dāsī and Harṣarāṇī Devī Dāsī, January 15, 1968)

So you should take it that your hospitalization is an opportunity of chanting Hare Kṛṣṇa mantra 24 hours. After all we are not this body so bodily disorders cannot hamper our advancement in Kṛṣṇa consciousness. So long the tongue is active we can chant. Even if the tongue is not active we can think of Kṛṣṇa. Someway or other if we can keep in touch with Kṛṣṇa that is our success of life.

(Letter to Cidānanda Dāsa, September 28, 1971)

Real Healthy Life is Kṛṣṇa Consciousness

Our healthy life is to go back to the spiritual world and serve Lord Kṛṣṇa there.

Prabhupāda: Now, healthy, what do you mean by healthy?
Father Tanner: Well, you know, you were saying it's what a man does that makes him that if he is pure here and now, then, and it's not his inside. It's his outside...
Prabhupāda: Our description of healthy life, healthy life is to become God conscious. That is healthy life. Otherwise do you think that an animal like elephant, very strong, does it mean that it is healthy? No.
Father Tanner: No, I would say an elephant can be healthy, my body can be healthy.
Prabhupāda: Well, that is temporary. Everyone is subjected to death. So you may be very strong, healthy, but you cannot avoid death.
Father Tanner: No, but then, then...
Prabhupāda: So, so therefore, ultimately, you become so-called healthy or not healthy, you'll die. That is the fact. So we do not want that kind of healthy life. Our proposition is that we go back to home back to Godhead and remain with God, eternally enjoying blissful life. This is our healthy life.

(Conversation with Father Tanner and other guests, London, July 11, 1973)

Spiritual Advancement Will Keep the Body Healthy

All energies come from the Supreme Lord. If you're Kṛṣṇa consciousness, all the energies that keep the body healthy will also be present.

Prabhupāda: Actually spiritual consciousness keeps the body fit. Just like in the body the spirit soul is there and the consciousness is also there, maybe polluted, but as soon as the spirit soul gives up this body, the body immediately begins to decompose. So the decomposition of the body is checked by the spiritual presence. So if you become advanced in spiritual consciousness there is no question of suffering from bodily disease.

(Lecture on Bhagavad-gītā 2.14, Mexico, February 14, 1975)

Entering that most sacred spot with his daughter and going near the sage, the first monarch, Svāyambhuva Manu, saw the sage sitting in his hermitage, having just propitiated the sacred fire by pouring oblations into it. His body shone most brilliantly; though he had engaged in austere penance for a long time, he was not emaciated, for the Lord had cast His affectionate sidelong glance upon him and he had also heard the nectar flowing from the moonlike words of the Lord. The sage was tall, his eyes were large, like the petals of a lotus, and he had matted locks on his head. He was clad in rags. Svāyambhuva Manu approached and saw him to be somewhat soiled, like an unpolished gem.

(Śrīmad-Bhāgavatam 3.21.45–47)

Here are some descriptions of a *brahmacārī-yogi*. In the morning, the first duty of a *brahmacārī* seeking spiritual elevation is *huta-hutāśana*, to offer sacrificial oblations to the Supreme Lord. Those engaged in *brahmacarya* cannot sleep until seven or nine o'clock in the morning. They must rise early in the morning, at least one and a half hours before the sun rises, and offer oblations, or in this age, they must chant the holy name of the Lord, Hare Kṛṣṇa. As referred to by Lord Caitanya, *kalau nāsty eva nāsty eva nāsty eva gatir anyathā*: there is no other alternative, no other alternative, no other alternative, in this age, to chanting the holy name of the Lord. The *brahmacārī* must rise early in the morning and, after placing himself, should chant the holy name of the Lord. From the very features of the sage, it appeared that he had undergone great austerities; that is the sign of one observing *brahmacarya*, the vow of celibacy. If one lives otherwise, it will be manifest in the lust visible in his face and body. The word *vidyotamānam* indicates that the *brahmacārī* feature showed in his body. That is the certificate that one has undergone great austerity in yoga. A drunkard or smoker or sex-monger can never be eligible to practice yoga. Generally yogis look very skinny because of their not being comfortably situated, but Kardama Muni was not emaciated, for he had seen the Supreme Personality of Godhead face to face. Here the word *snigdhāpāṅgāvalokanāt* means that he was fortunate enough to see the Supreme Lord face to face. He looked healthy because he had directly received the nectarean sound vibrations from the lotus lips of the Personality of Godhead. Similarly, one who hears the transcendental sound vibration of the holy name of the Lord, Hare Kṛṣṇa, also improves in health. We have actually seen that many *brahmacārīs* and *gṛhasthas* connected with the International Society for Kṛṣṇa Consciousness have improved in health, and a luster has come to their faces. It is essential that a *brahmacārī* engaged in spiritual advancement look very healthy and lustrous.

(Śrīmad-Bhāgavatam 3.21.45–47, purport)

Bob: I'd like to ask you just something I talked with devotees about—medicine. I walked to the river with some devotees today. I have a cold, so I said I shouldn't go in the water. Some felt I should because it is the Ganges, and some said I shouldn't because I have a cold, and we were talking, and I don't understand. Do we get sick because of our bad actions in the past?
Śrīla Prabhupāda: Yes, that's a fact.
Bob: But when one...
Śrīla Prabhupāda: Any kind of distress we suffer is due to our impious activities in the past.
Bob: But when someone is removed from karmic influence...
Śrīla Prabhupāda: Yes?
Bob: ... does he still get sick?
Śrīla Prabhupāda: No. Even if he gets sick, that is very temporary. For instance, this fan is moving. If you disconnect the electric power, then the fan will move for a moment. That movement is not due to the electric current. That is force—what is it called, physically, this force?
Śyāmasundara: Momentum.
Śrīla Prabhupāda: Momentum. But as soon as it stops, no more movement. Similarly, even if a devotee who has surrendered to Kṛṣṇa is suffering from material consequences, that is temporary. Therefore, a devotee does not take any material miseries as miseries. He takes them as Kṛṣṇa's, God's, mercy.
Bob: A perfected soul, a devotee, a pure devotee...
Śrīla Prabhupāda: A perfected soul is one who engages twenty-four hours a day in Kṛṣṇa consciousness. That is perfection. That is a transcendental position. Perfection means to engage in one's original consciousness. That is perfection. That is stated in *Bhagavad-gītā:*

sve sve karmaṇy abhirataḥ
saṁsiddhiṁ labhate naraḥ
[Bg. 18.45]

"By following his qualities of work, every man can become perfect." Complete perfection. *Saṁsiddhi. Siddhi* is perfection. That is Brahman realization, spiritual realization. And *saṁsiddhi* means devotion, which comes after Brahman realization.

Bob: Could you just say that last thing again please?

Śrīla Prabhupāda: *Saṁsiddhi.*

Bob: Yes.

Śrīla Prabhupāda: *Sam* means complete.

Bob: Yes.

Śrīla Prabhupāda: And *siddhi* means perfection. In the *Bhagavad-gītā* it is stated that one who goes back home, back to Godhead, has attained the complete perfection. So perfection comes when one realizes that he is not this body; he is spirit soul. *Brahmā-bhūta* [SB 4.30.20]—that is called Brahman realization. That is perfection. And *saṁsiddhi* comes after Brahman realization, when one engages in devotional service. Therefore if one is already engaged in devotional service, it is to be understood that Brahman realization is there. Therefore it is called *saṁsiddhi.*

Bob: I ask you this very humbly, but do you feel diseases and sickness?

Śrīla Prabhupāda: Hm-m?

Bob: Do you personally feel disease and sickness?

Śrīla Prabhupāda: Yes.

Bob: Is this a result of your past karma?

Śrīla Prabhupāda: Yes.

Bob: So one in this material world never escapes his karma completely?

Śrīla Prabhupāda: Yes, he escapes. No more karma for a devotee. No more karmic reaction.

Bob: But you must be the best devotee.

Śrīla Prabhupāda: Hm-m... No, I don't consider myself the best devotee. I am the lowest.

Bob: No!

Śrīla Prabhupāda: You are the best devotee.

Bob: [Laughs.] Oh, no, no! But, see, you say—what you say... always seems right.

Śrīla Prabhupāda: Yes.

Bob: Then you must be the best devotee.
Śrīla Prabhupāda: The thing is that even the best devotee, when he preaches, comes to the second-class platform of a devotee.
Bob: What would the best devotee be doing?
Śrīla Prabhupāda: The best devotee does not preach.
Bob: What does he do?
Śrīla Prabhupāda: He sees that there is no need of preaching. For him, everyone is a devotee. [Bob laughs heartily] Yes, he sees no more nondevotees—all devotees. He is called an *uttama-adhikārī*. But while I am preaching, how can I say I am the best devotee? Just like Rādhārāṇī—She does not see anyone as a nondevotee. Therefore we try to approach Rādhārāṇī.
Bob: Who is this?
Śrīla Prabhupāda: Rādhārāṇī, Kṛṣṇa's consort.
Bob: Ah.
Śrīla Prabhupāda: If anyone approaches Rādhārāṇī, She recommends to Kṛṣṇa, "Here is the best devotee. He is better than Me," and Kṛṣṇa cannot refuse him. That is the best devotee. But it is not to be imitated: "I have become the best devotee."

īśvare tad-adhīneṣu
bāliśeṣu dviṣatsu ca
prema-maitrī-kṛpopekṣā
yaḥ karoti sa madhyamaḥ
(SB 11.2.46)

A second-class devotee has the vision that some are envious of God, but this is not the vision of the best devotee. The best devotee sees, "Nobody is envious of God. Everyone is better than me." Just like *Caitanya-caritāmṛta's* author, Kṛṣṇadāsa Kavirāja. He says, "I am lower than the worm in the stool."
Bob: Who is saying this?
Śrīla Prabhupāda: Kṛṣṇadāsa Kavirāja, the author of *Caitanya-caritāmṛta*: *purīṣera kīṭa haite muñi se laghiṣṭha* [Cc. Ādi 5.205]. He is not making a show. He is feeling like that. "I am the lowest. Everyone is best, but I am the lowest. Everyone is engaged in Kṛṣṇa's service. I am not engaged." Caitanya Mahāprabhu said, "Oh, I have not a pinch of devotion to Kṛṣṇa. I cry to make a show. If I had been a devotee of Kṛṣṇa, I would have died long ago. But I am living. That is the proof that I do not love Kṛṣṇa."

That is the vision of the best devotee. He is so much absorbed in Kṛṣṇa's love that he says, "Everything is going on, but I am the lowest. Therefore I cannot see God." That is the best devotee.

Bob: So a devotee must work for everybody's liberation?

Śrīla Prabhupāda: Yes. A devotee must work under the direction of a bona fide spiritual master, not imitate the best devotee.

Bob: Excuse me?

Śrīla Prabhupāda: One should not imitate the best devotee.

Bob: Imitate. Oh. I see.

Śyāmasundara: One time you said that sometimes you feel sickness or pain due to the sinful activities of your devotees. Can sometimes disease be due to that? Caused by that?

Śrīla Prabhupāda: You see, Kṛṣṇa says:

ahaṁ tvāṁ sarva-pāpebhyo
mokṣayiṣyāmi mā śucaḥ
[Bg. 18.66]

"I will deliver you from all sinful reaction. Do not fear." So Kṛṣṇa is so powerful that He can immediately take up all the sins of others and immediately make them right. But when a living entity plays the part on behalf of Kṛṣṇa, he also takes the responsibility for the sinful activities of his devotees. Therefore to become a guru is not an easy task. You see? He has to take all the poisons and absorb them. So sometimes—because he is not Kṛṣṇa—sometimes there is some trouble. Therefore Caitanya Mahāprabhu has forbidden, "Don't make many *Śiṣyas*, many disciples." But for preaching work we have to accept many disciples—for expanding preaching—even if we suffer. That's a fact. The spiritual master has to take the responsibility for all the sinful activities of his disciples. Therefore to make many disciples is a risky job unless one is able to assimilate all the sins.

vāñchā-kalpa-tarubhyaś ca
kṛpā-sindhubhya eva ca
patitānāṁ pāvanebhyo
vaiṣṇavebhyo namo namaḥ

["I offer my respectful obeisances unto all the Vaiṣṇava devotees of the Lord. They are just like desire trees who can fulfill the desires of everyone, and they are full of compassion for the fallen conditioned souls."] He takes responsibility for all the fallen souls. That idea is also in the Bible.

Jesus Christ took all the sinful reactions of the people and sacrificed his life. That is the responsibility of a spiritual master. Because Kṛṣṇa is Kṛṣṇa, He is *apāpa-viddha*—He cannot be attacked by sinful reactions. But a living entity is sometimes subjected to their influence because he is so small. Big fire, small fire. If you put some big thing in a small fire, the fire itself may be extinguished. But in a big fire, whatever you put in is all right. The big fire can consume anything.

Bob: Christ's suffering was of that nature?

Śrīla Prabhupāda: Mm-m?

Bob: Was Christ's suffering—

Śrīla Prabhupāda: That I have already explained. He took the sinful reactions of all the people. Therefore he suffered.

Bob: I see.

Śrīla Prabhupāda: He said—that is in the Bible—that he took all the sinful reactions of the people and sacrificed his life. But these Christian people have made it a law for Christ to suffer while they do all nonsense. [Bob gives a short laugh.] Such great fools they are! They have let Jesus Christ make a contract for taking all their sinful reactions so they can go on with all nonsense. That is their religion. Christ was so magnanimous that he took all their sins and suffered, but that does not induce them to stop all these sins. They have not come to that sense. They have taken it very easily. "Let Lord Jesus Christ suffer, and we'll do all nonsense." Is it not?

Bob: It is so.

Śrīla Prabhupāda: They should have been ashamed: "Lord Jesus Christ suffered for us, but we are continuing the sinful activities." He told everyone, "Thou shalt not kill," but they are indulging in killing, thinking, "Lord Jesus Christ will excuse us and take all the sinful reactions." This is going on. We should be very much cautious: "For my sinful actions my spiritual master will suffer, so I'll not commit even a pinch of sinful activities." That is the duty of the disciple. After initiation, all sinful reaction is finished. Now if he again commits sinful activities, his spiritual master has to suffer. A disciple should be sympathetic and consider this. "For my sinful activities, my spiritual master will suffer." If the spiritual master is attacked by some disease, it is due to the sinful activities of others. "Don't make many disciples." But we do it because we are preaching. Never mind—let us suffer—still we shall accept them.

Therefore your question was—when I suffer is it due to my past misdeeds? Was it not? That is my misdeed—that I accepted some disciples who are nonsense. That is my misdeed.

Bob: This happens on occasions?

Śrīla Prabhupāda: Yes. This is sure to happen because we are accepting so many men. It is the duty of the disciples to be cautious. "My spiritual master has saved me. I should not put him again into suffering." When the spiritual master is in suffering, Kṛṣṇa saves him. Kṛṣṇa thinks, "Oh, he has taken so much responsibility for delivering a fallen person." So Kṛṣṇa is there.

kaunteya pratijānīhi
na me bhaktaḥ praṇaśyati
[Bg. 9.31]

["O son of Kuntī, declare it boldly that My devotee never perishes."] Because the spiritual master takes the risk on account of Kṛṣṇa.

Bob: Your suffering is not the same kind of pain...

Śrīla Prabhupāda: No, it is not due to karma. The pain is there sometimes, so that the disciples may know, "Due to our sinful activities, our spiritual master is suffering."

Bob: You look very well now.

Śrīla Prabhupāda: I am always well... in the sense that even if there is suffering, I know Kṛṣṇa will protect me. But this suffering is not due to my sinful activities.

Bob: But let us say when I—in the town I live in, I take boiled water because some of the water has disease in it. Now, why should I drink boiled water if I have been good enough not to get a disease? Then I may drink any water. And if I have been not acting properly. then I shall get disease anyway.

Śrīla Prabhupāda: So long as you are in the material world, you cannot neglect physical laws. Suppose you go to a jungle and there is a tiger. It is known that it will attack you, so why should you voluntarily go and be attacked? It is not that a devotee should take physical risk so long as he has a physical body. It is not a challenge to the physical laws: "I have become a devotee. I challenge everything." That is foolishness.

anāsaktasya viṣayān
yathārham upayuñjataḥ

nirbandhaḥ kṛṣṇa-sambandhe
yuktaṁ vairāgyam ucyate
(Bhakti-rasāmṛta-sindhu 1.2.255)

The devotee is advised to accept the necessities of life without attachment. He'll take boiled water, but if boiled water is not available, does it mean he will not drink water? If it is not available, he will drink ordinary water. We take Kṛṣṇa *prasāda*, but while touring, sometimes we have to take some food in a hotel. Because one is a devotee, should he think, "I will not take any foodstuffs from the hotel. I shall starve"? If I starve, then I will be weak and will not be able to preach. (*Perfect Questions Perfect Answers, Chapter* 6)

Relief from Bodily and Spiritual Diseases

Birth, disease, old age, and death are our real problems, and the Kṛṣṇa consciousness movement has the cure for them.

As Murāri Gupta treated his patients, by his mercy both their bodily and spiritual diseases subsided.

(Caitanya-caritāmṛta, Adi-līlā 10.51)

Murāri Gupta could treat both bodily and spiritual disease because he was a physician by profession and a great devotee of the Lord in terms of spiritual advancement. This is an example of service to humanity. Everyone should know that there are two kinds of diseases in human society. One disease, which is called *ādhyātmika*, or material disease, pertains to the body, but the main disease is spiritual.

The living entity is eternal, but somehow or other, when in contact with the material energy, he is subjected to the repetition of birth, death, old age and disease. The physicians of the modern day should learn from Murāri Gupta. Although modern philanthropic physicians open gigantic hospitals, there are no hospitals to cure the material disease of the spirit soul. The Kṛṣṇa consciousness movement has taken up the mission of curing this disease, but people are not very appreciative because they do not know what this disease is. A diseased person needs both proper medicine and a proper diet, and therefore the Kṛṣṇa consciousness movement supplies materially stricken people with the medicine of the chanting of the holy name, or the Hare Kṛṣṇa *mahā-mantra*, and the diet of *prasādam*. There are many hospitals and medical clinics to cure bodily diseases, but there are no such hospitals to cure the material disease of the spirit soul. The centers of the Kṛṣṇa consciousness movement are the only established hospitals that can cure man of birth, death, old age and disease.

(Caitanya-caritāmṛta, Adi-līlā 10.51, purport)

He brought up the same point again at the end of his *Śrīmad-Bhāgavatam* lecture. He told us that the disease of everyone in the material world is the desire to be a master. Whether a person has charge of one or two family members or the entire universe like Lord Brahmā, the disease is the same. So when people come to our Kṛṣṇa conscious Society, the leaders have to be alert to see to the treatment of this disease.

(Transcendental Diary, Vol. 1, Chap. 9, March 4, 1976)

Śrī G. Gopāla Reddy, the president of the local Rotary Club, also accompanied Śrīla Prabhupāda on the morning walk. He is the secretary of a committee that Mahāṁsa Swami has formed for the new temple. The committee has been very active in making new ISKCON life members and obtaining pledges for construction work. Prabhupāda was happy to see him and thanked him for his efforts. Upon noticing a colony of *bhaṅgis*, or "untouchables," Mr. Reddy mentioned that the government was distributing land to them. He asked whether ISKCON was engaged in any sort of social welfare work, because many people have asked him what our Society did to benefit others.

Prabhupāda replied by asking him what he considered the best social welfare.

When Mr. Reddy said serving the poor and the natives, Prabhupāda told him, "Everyone is poor. Who is rich? First of all find out: Who is rich?" Śrīla Prabhupāda went on to explain how everyone is poor because each of us must suffer disease, old age, and death. Adjustment of a person's material condition can be done by anyone, but ISKCON was established for a different purpose. "These things are being done by so many other people, and we are doing something which is ultimate. The hospital gives some medicine when there is some disease, but that does not mean there will be no disease. Can they guarantee that, 'I give you this medicine – no more disease?' We are giving that medicine – that no more disease. That is the best social work. As soon as you give up this body – *tyaktvā dehaṁ punar janma naiti* – you'll have no more birth. And if you have no more birth, there will be no more death. And if you have no more birth, then there will be no more disease. This is our prescription. *Tyaktvā dehaṁ punar janma naiti mām eti.* Not that he is finished; he goes back to home, back to Godhead. This is our program."

(Transcendental Diary, Vol. 1, Chap. 7, January 7, 1976)

Real Hospital

The Kṛṣṇa consciousness movement is the real hospital to cure people from the repetition of birth and death.

It is not uncommon in India for a man to give up all material engagements, to leave his home and family and take the renounced order, *sannyasa*, and after meditating for some while, begin doing philanthropic work by opening some hospitals or engaging in politics. The hospital-making business is being conducted by the government; it is the duty of a *sannyāsī* to make hospitals whereby people can actually get rid of their material bodies, not patch them up. But for want of knowing what real spiritual activity is, we take up material activities.

(Rāja-Vidyā, Chapter 7)

Śrīla Prabhupāda is feeling stronger, and the swelling in his body has gone down because of the diuretic pills Dr. Patel supplied yesterday. But Prabhupāda didn't take all the pills prescribed. After taking a half tablet, as soon as he got the desired effect, he stopped taking the medication.

He resumed his morning exercise, walking down to Juhu Beach as usual.

Prabhupāda asked Saurabha about a dentist interested in opening a clinic in the new temple compound. Saurabha explained that the man had seen the floor plan, which includes a room for medical use, and immediately proposed that he use it to give free treatment to the devotees.

Prabhupāda did not approve. "No, there will be no medical service in the building."

Lokanātha Swami asked if medical facilities should be set up on another part of the land.

Prabhupāda replied, "That we shall do at our convenience. It is not very urgent. When there is spare room, then. Medical service is to cure the material disease, this temporary headache and stomachache. There are so many medical services for these things, but where is the medical service for curing *bhava-roga*, material disease? That is wanted. Medical service does not give any guarantee that there will be no more disease. Our service is to guarantee that there will be no more birth, death, old age, and disease. That is the difference."

Pausing for a moment, he recalled his recent trip to Africa. "In Mauritius I was suffering so much from dental pain. I never went to the dentist; I invented my medicine and it cured."

Everyone smiled in admiration. Prabhupāda seems to know nearly everything. He was referring to his own toothpaste recipe: a combination of ground mustard seed, salt, calcium carbonate, eucalyptus oil, camphor, menthol, and oil of wintergreen. Many devotees are now eagerly making it for themselves, and Prabhupāda asked if they like it.

He grinned when Harikeśa assured him, "Oh yes! The best!" Lokanātha Swami voiced what we all felt, "You are perfect in all respects. You are your own doctor."

Prabhupāda humbly responded, "I am not doctor, but I created many doctors."

(Transcendental Diary, Vol. 1, Chap. 4, December 23, 1975)

Devotees Should Look After the Other Devotees

Ask Them What They Need

Devotees who are leaders should supply whatever the devotees under their care need, even if they do not ask for it.

Prabhupāda: Mm. (pause) So you don't require covering? This girl? This cloth is sufficient? What you think? Why you have no covering? Mm? You

do not require cloth?
Kulādri: It is warm for us Śrīla Prabhupāda.
Prabhupāda: No, if they require, there must be supply. You must ask them what they need and provide them because they do not say you'll also keep silent. That's not good. Every month they must be asked what they need. Necessities, they must be supplied. We have already discussed this point, the women; they require protection, children, and women.

(Conversation, New Vrindaban, June 26, 1976)

GBC's Concern

GBC members should handle the needs of devotees according to what is practical.

Your write that our society should provide some medical facility, insurance or personnel to handle devotees who become chronically ill and thus ostracized from our society. Of course this kind of management of affairs is better handled by the GBC which I have created for this purpose, I cannot be expected to handle problems of this sort while at the same time writing my books.

First of all, there is no question of a devotee becoming ostracized because he has become ill, nor do I think this is being widely practiced. Who has been ostracized? One of the symptoms of a devotee is that he is kind, so if our Godbrother becomes ill it is our duty to help him get the proper medicine and treatment so that he can recover. Of course, this kind of management of affairs is better handled by the GBC which I have created for this purpose.

Recently our Girirāja became chronically ill in India and had to return to the U.S. for proper medical treatment. There, in our Los Angeles center, he was given his own room and was able to recuperate comfortably, and now he has returned to his full duties in Bombay. Now Tamāl Kṛṣṇa Gosvāmī has just had a successful hernia operation which was arranged free of charge at one of the most modern hospitals, and there is also a girl devotee undergoing operation there also. Tamāl Kṛṣṇa is now living in a room at our temple; the devotees see that he gets all facility, a hospital bed, proper *prasādam*, and personal care and visiting.

So there is no question of ill-treating our own Godbrothers simply because they are sick, nor should you allow such neglect to go on. So long we have this material body there will be sickness, but we have to remain on the transcendental platform nevertheless.

As far as a centralized medical plan for the whole society, no such plan or facility or insurance has seemed practical as yet. The best thing is to work it out locally, try to find the services of a free medical facility in Seattle, or some way that sick devotees can be cared for; that is your responsibility. I think further questions of this sort can be handled by the GBC.

(Letter to Śukadeva Dāsa, April 5, 1974)

Sympathetic

Devotees should show care and concern for sick devotees and should do everything necessary to help them.

We should be very much sympathetic. If some of our fellow men fall sick, we must take care of him, give help him. Because, after all, we have got this body. Sometimes we may fall sick. So one, we should be sympathetic.

(Lecture on Śrīmad-Bhāgavatam 2.3.13,
Los Angeles, May 30, 1972)

Prabhupāda visited Geneva in 1974, and Līlāvatī dāsī arrived there to type for him, but she had contracted hepatitis and soon had to go into the hospital. Three days after his arrival, Prabhupāda called for the temple president, Guru Gaurāṅga, and asked him where Līlāvatī was. He was told that she was in the hospital. Prabhupāda then asked if anyone had gone to see her, and Guru Gaurāṅga explained that everyone had been so busy that no one had thought to go. We shall go see Līlāvatī. Make all preparation, Prabhupāda said.

Guru Gaurāṅga immediately set about readying the car and devotees, and he made arrangements for *prasādam*. When everything was ready, he told Prabhupāda. Prabhupāda said, Very good, and told them all to go to see Līlāvatī.

Prabhupāda himself stayed behind, but almost everyone else in the temple went to see Līlāvatī, who became very much enlivened by the care and concern which Prabhupāda was showing her.

(Śrīla Prabhupāda Nectar, Vol. 5, No. 10)

During the morning Śrīla Prabhupāda noticed I was limping because of a boil forming on my leg. Later, while talking with Jayapatāka Mahārāja, he called me in and told me to show him the boil. Prabhupāda was so thoughtful that he asked Jayapatāka to go out and buy some medicine to heal the boil. I was somewhat embarrassed that a *sannyāsī* should be running an errand on my behalf, but Prabhupāda was more concerned to see that it was cured. Like a loving father, he always takes time to see that we are properly looked after, especially concerning our health.

(Transcendental Diary, Vol. 1, Chap. 8, January 13, 1976)

Chapter 3
Maintaining Health

Diet

Basis of All Food

You only need grains, ghee, yogurt, and milk to prepare nutritious food. Therefore, if there are land and cows, the economic problem of producing grains and milk can be solved. Other foods, such as fruit, can be useful but are not necessary.

Anna, *ghṛta*, *dadhi* and *dugdha* are food grains, ghee, yogurt and milk. Actually these are the basis of all food. Vegetables and fruits are subsidiary. Hundreds and thousands of recipes can be made out of grains, vegetables, ghee, milk and yogurt. The food offered to *Gopala* in the Annakūṭa ceremony contained only these five ingredients. Only demoniac people are attracted to other types of food, which we will not even mention in this connection. We should understand that in order to prepare nutritious food, we require only grains, ghee, yogurt and milk. We cannot offer anything else to the Deity. The Vaiṣṇava, the perfect human being, does not accept anything not offered to the Deity. People are often frustrated with national food policies, but from the Vedic scriptures we find that if there are sufficient cows and grains, the entire food problem is solved. The *vaiśya* (people engaged in agriculture and commerce) are therefore recommended in *Bhagavad-gītā* to produce grains and give protection to cows. Cows are the most important animal because they produce the miracle food, milk, from which we can prepare ghee and yogurt.

The perfection of human civilization depends on Kṛṣṇa consciousness, which recommends Deity worship. Preparations made from vegetables, grains, milk, ghee and yogurt are offered to the Deity and then distributed. Here we can see the difference between the East and the West. The people who came to see the Deity of *Gopala* brought all kinds of food to offer the Deity. They brought all the food they had in stock, and they came before the Deity not only to accept *prasāda* for themselves, but to distribute it to others. The Kṛṣṇa consciousness movement vigorously approves this practice of preparing food, offering it to the Deity, and distributing it to the general population. This activity should be extended universally to stop sinful eating habits as well as other behavior befitting only demons. A demoniac civilization will never bring peace within the world.

Since eating is the first necessity in human society, those engaged in solving the problems of preparing and distributing food should take lessons from Mādhavendra Purī and execute the Annakūṭa ceremony. When the people take to eating only prasāda offered to the Deity, all the demons will be turned into Vaiṣṇavas. When the people are Kṛṣṇa conscious, naturally the government will be so also. A Kṛṣṇa conscious man is always a very liberal well-wisher of everyone. When such men head the government, the people will certainly be sinless. They will no longer be disturbing demons. It is then and then only that a peaceful condition can prevail in society.

(Caitanya-caritāmṛta, Madhya-līlā 4.93, purport)

Mahāvīra came to see Śrīla Prabhupāda about the temple *prasādam*. He explained with some consternation that several devotees are complaining because the daily fare is *kichuḍi* [food prepared from rice and lentils] and *chapattis* for breakfast, and rice, *dāl* and *chapattis* for lunch, with an occasional *subji*. Their main complaint seems to be about the lack of variety and the absence of fruit. Being new to India and also being satisfied himself with the simple menu, Mahāvīra wasn't sure what the standard should be, so he requested that Prabhupāda advise him.

Prabhupāda wasn't too concerned. He told him, "Humans are

grain eaters. If they want to eat fruit, then let them just eat fruit only. Otherwise, just leave it the way it is."

(Transcendental Diary, Vol. 5, Chap. 3, November 19, 1976)

Breakfast for Puṣṭa Kṛṣṇa Mahārāja and myself consists of fresh mangoes, pineapples and *halavā* (sweet made with sugar, butter, and farina). Śrīla Prabhupāda is also enjoying the fresh ripe fruits, freely available in the neighborhood. Remarking on the delicious mangoes he said that their juice should be boiled down and then dried in trays in the sun. He explained that this dried pulp can be stored for years, and when eaten with ground rice and milk is both palatable and nutritious.

(Transcendental Diary, Vol. 2, Chap. 4, May 8,, 1976)

Diet for a Sick Devotee

When a devotee is sick, sometimes a special diet is necessary.

Regarding the diet which the doctors are giving you, it is all right if you do not take milk for some time. Vegetables will do.

(Letter to Baradrāja Dāsa, October 21, 1969)

Because his digestion is poor and he is suffering from excess mucus, Prabhupāda has been adjusting his diet. His liver is not functioning properly, and his digestion is not good. He has stopped taking evening *prasādam*. For breakfast he is eating only fruits, and for lunch he has a variety of vegetable preparations, but no *dāl* or rice.

Today he decided to take his evening milk in the form of milk sweets like *rasagullās* or *sandeśa* made with *gur*, a local form of brown sugar made from boiled-down cane juice. He reasoned that the sugar would be good for his liver and the solid milk would give him strength to work on his books throughout the night. (As a liquid, milk is too difficult for him to digest.)

(Transcendental Diary, Vol. 1, Chap. 9, February 8, 1976)

Eat Nice Nutritious Food

Eat nice nutritious food and be Kṛṣṇa conscious.

Regarding your letter asking me permission for taking *prasādam* comprising fruits, nuts, milk products and green leafy vegetables—if the__to your health for rendering service to Kṛṣṇa with more energy then you must take such *prasāda* instead of cooked food. If required you can take raw cereals soaked in water overnight—that is also good. The thing is you must accept such food as will keep you fit. Not more nor less, that is the injunction of Lord Kṛṣṇa in the *Bhagavad-gītā*. Hope you are well.

(Letter to Dayānanda Dāsa, March 23, 1969)

Prabhupāda: We have no other business. We want to see people live, eating very nicely nutritious food, keeping good health. But unnecessarily artificial things, bothering, that we don't want. Keep your health very nice, live for as many years as possible, and be Kṛṣṇa conscious. Then, next life, you go back to home, back to Godhead, permanent life. *Yad gatvā na nivartante [Bg 15.6]*. This we want to give. There is no cheating. There is no politics, no personal ambition fulfilling. This is our mission.

(Conversation, May 27, 1977)

For breakfast Prabhupāda again had some of the season's first produce, some sugar-cane juice from our own fields. He is very happy to see our men using the land to grow foodstuff. The *dāl* (soup made from lentils) we drink daily is home-grown, and the *capātīs* are made from our own wheat.

(Transcendental Diary, Vol. 1, Chap. 9, January 19, 1976)

Raw Diet

When I first moved into the temple, I ate whatever *prasāda* was served. Then I became Prabhupāda's cook, so I had a kitchen, and I could prepare what I wanted. I had come from a Southern California raw-food background, and I started eating salads and fruits and simple food but

I wanted to make sure that I was not going against what Prabhupāda wanted. One day I decided to ask him about a raw diet as opposed to taking *prasāda*. He said, "Actually, a raw diet is the best diet for Kṛṣṇa consciousness. It's simple. It keeps your body healthy and clear. We don't tell the masses about it, because most people can't follow it, and we don't want them to get distracted from Kṛṣṇa. But if you can do it, it's the best diet for your Kṛṣṇa consciousness."

(Interview with Nanda Kumar Dāsa)

There was a time when Prabhupāda was having some physical challenges. I had come from a health-food background, and there was a doctor in India that also said, "Prabhupāda should eat raw food." I thought, "Yes, yes, this is good. I can do that. I can make raw-food preparations." I told Prabhupāda, "This person has suggested eating a very light diet without ghee." Prabhupāda said, "I will do this." I thought, "This is going to be really good. Prabhupāda's health will become strong." I prepared one meal like that, and Prabhupāda said, "This is very good." The next morning—his morning *prasāda* was almost always simple things like fruits and milk—I said, "What would you like for lunch?" Prabhupāda said, "Dahl, rice, *chapatis*, *halavā*." I asked him about the raw diet. He said, "Since I was a child, I have always loved *prasādam*, and I'm not going to give it up now. I will eat *prasādam*, and Kṛṣṇa will protect me."

(Interview with Nanda Kumar Dāsa)

Prasāda and Preaching

To maximize preaching, a devotee can alter his or her diet and adjust the number of meals he or she takes.

So you are all intelligent boys, so you should judge the desire of my Guru Mahārāja (spiritual master) and help me in that way. Regarding the temple management, one man can be left behind, while the others go out, to take care of the Deity. And, you can come home at night and take *prasādam* sumptuously. Once eating sumptuously is enough to maintain body and soul together. In the daytime you may not take, and at night you can take. As a matter of fact, a devotee may take only once in a day either in the day or night, and whenever you eat, you must first offer. But I do not mean you should neglect temple life. Do not misunderstand this. But, one man can remain, and so far the other devotees are concerned, they can eat once in the day or night, after having *kīrtana*, then six hours of sound sleep, and this will maintain their health properly.

(Letter to Śrī Govinda Dāsa, December 6, 1974)

Prabhupāda focused once more on book distribution. He was eager for more association with Prabhaviṣṇu and Prabhaviṣṇu was eager for his. Prabhupāda was pleased to hear that both the books and his disciples were being well received wherever they went. He advised Prabhaviṣṇu how to stay fit for his service. "Keep your health nice, because Indian climate sometimes does not suit. Eat simple things. Fruits, vegetables. Don't be miser in the matter of…But don't eat voraciously. Eat sufficiently, nutritious. Vegetable, fruits, very innocent, little milk. That's all."

His next suggestion made Prabhaviṣṇu raise his eyebrows and laugh a little in mild apprehension and surprise. "Even if you don't eat these food grains, that is preferred, better. Vegetable and fruits and milk, that is sufficient nutritious. There is no question of disease. But for our tongue taste we eat so many cooked food, but if we eat vegetables, boiled vegetables and fruits and milk, ah, it is sufficient. Ekādaśī, daily Ekādaśī. And these peanuts, a few grains. Not much. That is also nice. Cashew, peanut, yes."

(Transcendental Diary, Vol. 4, Chap. 3, August 22, 1976)

Eat Only Prasāda, Food Offered to Lord Kṛṣṇa

On another morning walk in Denver, Tamāl Kṛṣṇa Gosvāmī told Prabhupāda that some of the devotees were reading books about health diets and were avoiding the *prasādam* offered to the Deity in the temple. Śrīla Prabhupāda immediately replied that this was not good. Fasting, he acknowledged, was good for health, but the devotees should not become weak. They should take *prasādam* and do their work.

When one of the devotees told Prabhupāda he got drowsy after eating heavily of grains and therefore preferred fruit, Prabhupāda said that was all right; fruit was offered to the Deity. When Yadubara said that in Los Angeles the families often cooked in their own homes instead of taking the *prasādam* of the Deity, Bhāvānanda Gosvāmī testified how wonderful it was at the Māyāpur festival when hundreds of devotees sat down and took *prasādam* together.

Prabhupāda: "Yes, what is the difficulty? *Capātīs*, rice, they are innocent foods. What is the difficulty?"
Harikeśa: "A lot of devotees are quoting you. They say there is no need to eat grains and that you said that grains were for the animals."
Prabhupāda: "But I am eating grains."
Harikeśa: "I tell them that."
Prabhupāda: "They say, 'Prabhupāda says.' Then you believe that."

Prabhupāda said that devotees should not listen to health advice if it resulted in their refusing to honor the Lord's *prasādam*.

Prabhupāda: "Therefore, follow taking *prasādam*. Let whatever may happen."
Tamāl Kṛṣṇa: "Let us die eating *prasādam*."
Prabhupāda: "Yes. [Laughter.] That is devotee. But we must prepare very first class foodstuffs. And then, where is the complaint, if it is first class?"

Returning from the walk, Śrīla Prabhupāda continued to discuss the topic in Śrīmad-Bhāgavatam class: "I was hearing that we are not taking prasādam-especially the *gṛhasthas*. No. That is not good. You should take *prasādam*." Prabhupāda described how *bhakti-yoga* begins with controlling the tongue-by chanting and by eating Kṛṣṇa-*prasādam*.

"So in our branches," he continued, "all the devotees take *prasādam* together. That is nice. Why we should not be liking to take *prasādam* in the temple? What is the fault? No, this is not good. Everyone should take *prasādam*... It is called *prasāda-sevā* [service], not prasādam enjoyment. *Prasādam* means giving service. *Prasādam* is as good as Kṛṣṇa and should be respected as good as Kṛṣṇa. So one must have faith that it is not material. Those who are attached to the Kṛṣṇa consciousness movement and are attached to the service, they should take *prasādam*—first—class *prasādam*. Everyone likes the taste of *prasādam*."

(Śrīla Prabhupāda–līlāmṛta, Chap. 46)

Tapasya and Detachment

We are suffering in this material world because our existence is not pure. Therefore, we have to accept some austerity (tapasya). Austerity means controlling your eating, sexuality, and other types of sense gratification. In this way, you can use your time to advance spiritually and purify your body and mind. Of course, the senses should be gratified as much as is required to maintain our health.

Tapasya means to undergo voluntarily some inconveniences of this body. Because we are accustomed to enjoy bodily senses, and *tapasya* means voluntarily to give up the idea of sense gratification. That is tapasya. Tapasya. Just like Ekādaśī. Ekādaśī, one day fasting, fortnight. That is also tapasya. Or fasting in some other auspicious day. That *tapasya* is good, even for health, and what to speak of advancing in Kṛṣṇa consciousness. So we should accept this *tapasya*. The *upavāsa* (fasting). There are many prescribed days for fasting. We should observe. And the preliminary *tapasya*, no illicit sex, no gambling, no intoxication, no..., no meat-eating... There may be some inconvenience, those who were accustomed to this practice, but we'll have to accept. *Tapo divyāṁ putrakā yena sattvaṁ Śuddhyet* [*Śrīmad-Bhāgavatam* 5.5.1]. If we want to purify our existence... At the present moment our existence is not purified, impure. Therefore we are suffering. Just like when one's physiological condition becomes infected, he suffers from fever and other symptoms of disease, similarly, we are suffering in this material world on account of this material body. If we want really happiness, then we must accept *tapasya*. *Tapasya* is required. Without *tapasya*, if you think that very easily... Or Without tapasya, I can get it simply by imagination, then you become *sahajiyā*, to take things very easily. No. *Tapasya*.

(Lecture on Bhagavad-gītā 7.9, Vṛndāvana, August 15, 1974)

A patient suffering from a particular type of malady is almost always inclined to accept eatables which are forbidden for him. The expert physician does not make any compromise with the patient by allowing him to take partially what he should not at all take.

(Śrīmad-Bhāgavatam 1.5.15, purport)

We can definitely see that to advance in Kṛṣṇa consciousness one must control his bodily weight. If one becomes too fat, it is to be assumed that he is not advancing spiritually. Śrīla Bhaktisiddhānta Sarasvatī Ṭhākura severely criticized his fat disciples. The idea is that one who intends to advance in Kṛṣṇa consciousness must not eat very much. Devotees used to go to forests, high hills or mountains on pilgrimages, but such severe austerities are not possible in these days. One should instead eat only *prasāda* and no more than required. According to the Vaiṣṇava calendar, there are many fasts, such as Ekādaśī and the appearance and disappearance days of God and His devotees. All of these are meant to decrease the fat within the body so that one will not sleep more than desired and will not become inactive and lazy. Overindulgence in food will cause a man to sleep more than required. This human form of life is meant for austerity, and austerity means controlling sex, food intake, etc. In this way time can be saved for spiritual activity, and one can purify himself both externally and internally. Thus both body and mind can be cleansed.

(Śrīmad-Bhāgavatam 4.28.35–36, purport)

He described the condition of taking repeated births in the material realm as a diseased condition, and said that the acceptance of *tapasya* is the way to stop this disease. Surveying his audience, he addressed his new disciples, calling their attention to the great responsibility they were about to accept. "So this initiation means, don't think that it is something official, ritualistic ceremony, and as soon as we get the initiation, now we have become perfect and whatever nonsense I like I can do. No, *tapasya* must continue. In order to purify yourself, your existence, you have to continue the *tapasya*: no illicit sex, no meat-eating, no gambling, no intoxication and chant Hare Kṛṣṇa. If you follow these five principles, then your existence will be purified, you'll understand Kṛṣṇa from the *Bhagavad-gītā*, you'll know what is the purpose of life. The purpose of life is to understand Kṛṣṇa. There is no other business in this human form of life but because we have given up Kṛṣṇa, we have invented so many occupational duties. So so-called occupational running here and there on motor car is not the end of life. There is something more for the human being; that is *divyā-jñāna* (spiritual knowledge).

"Why shall I purify my existence? Because you want happiness. That is your desire. So you'll get *Brahmā-saukhyaṁ*, the greatest happiness which will never end. If you purify your existence by *tapasya* then you will be happy eternally. There will be no end. Here in this material world any happiness is temporary. Either for five minutes or five days or five years or five hundred years or five millions of years, it will end. But if you purify your existence, then the happiness will never end. *Tapo divyaṁ putrakā yena sattvaṁ Śuddhyed yasmād Brahmā-saukhyaṁ tv anantam. Anantam* means unlimited. It is very serious thing, and it is offered to the human being. So anyone can take advantage of this opportunity and make his life successful. Thank you very much."

(Transcendental Diary, Vol. 2, Chap. 7, June 18, 1976)

After taking breakfast Prabhupāda slept until noon. His face is now badly swollen and he has a severe toothache, but he refuses to visit a dentist. Better let it fall out by itself, he said, because a dentist will want to extract all of them. He simply sucks an occasional clove to help deaden the pain. It is yet another amazing display of his bodily detachment. Any ordinary man would be in agony, completely disturbed mentally, and complaining all the time. But Prabhupāda sits quietly and tolerates it without so much as a murmur.

(Transcendental Diary, Vol. 2, Chap. 7, June 18, 1976)

Prabhupāda is always concerned about our welfare – not just philosophically, but in many practical ways as well. For example, this morning was very cold; winter is really setting in. He remarked about it on his walk and then asked if the devotees are getting ghee on their *capātīs*. Akṣayānanda Swami replied that only the guests are given some because it's expensive and not necessary for the devotees.

But Prabhupāda disagreed. He said that it is necessary in this season. In the cold weather the devotees must have a little extra ghee and grains. He recommended a mix of *channa* and *urad dāls* as being both palatable and beneficial – not too little and not too much. "Unnecessary *vairāgya*," he said, "there is no need. We don't approve that. *Yuktāhāra-vihārasya*. What you require for keeping health – but not to eat too much. But what is absolutely required must be done."

(Transcendental Diary, Vol. 1, Chap. 2, December 8, 1975)

How Much to Eat

Satisfy the body's demands according to necessity, but not more than that. And don't completely fill up the stomach with food, but leave room for air and water.

If you are elephant you eat hundred pounds, but if you ant you eat one grain. Don't eat hundred pounds imitating the elephant. You see? God has given food to the elephant and to the ant. But if you are actually elephant then you eat like elephant. But if you are ant, don't eat like elephant, then you'll be in trouble. So here it is said, There is no possibility of one's becoming a yogi O Arjuna, if one eats too much or eats too little. Very nice program. Don't eat too little. You eat whatever you require. But don't eat more. Similarly don't sleep more. If you can keep your health perfect, but try to reduce it.

(Lecture on Bhagavad-gītā 6.16.24, Los Angeles, February 17, 1969)

By keeping regular habits and eating simple food, any man can maintain his health. Overeating, over-sense gratification, overdependence on another's mercy, and artificial standards of living sap the very vitality of human energy. Therefore the duration of life is shortened.

(*Śrīmad*-Bhāgavatam *1.1.10, purport)*

One should cease performing conventional religious practices and should be attracted to those which lead to salvation. One should eat very frugally and should always remain secluded so that he can achieve the highest perfection of life.

(*Śrīmad*-Bhāgavatam *3.28.3)*

The next important phrase is *mita-medhyādanam*, which means that one should eat very frugally. It is recommended in the Vedic literatures that a *yogi* eat only half what he desires according to his hunger. If one is so hungry that he could devour one pound of foodstuffs, then instead of eating one pound, he should consume only half a pound and supplement this with four ounces of water; one fourth of the stomach should be left empty for passage of air in the stomach. If one eats in this manner, he will avoid indigestion and disease. The *yogi* should eat in this way, as recommended in the *Śrīmad*-Bhāgavatam and all other standard scriptures.

(*Śrīmad*-Bhāgavatam *3.28.3, purport)*

Avoid Overeating

Sometimes overeating is the cause of sickness.

Poor people, they do not know what is their self-interest, what is the aim of life. Therefore Vyāsadeva he is called *vidvāṁs. Vidvāṁs* means very learned. He has compiled the *Śāstra. Anartha*, unnecessarily want. Wants we have increased.

Now we, instead of wasting our time for increasing our unnecessary needs of life, we shall be satisfied with the bare necessities of life. Eating, sleeping, mating, we can minimize it. But don't, we don't say that you starve, you keep your body uncomfortably, and then fall sick, and then your Kṛṣṇa conscious business is hampered.

No. *Yavad-artha prayojana. Anāsaktasya viṣayān.* Don't be attached to sense gratification. Satisfy senses as little as possible, which is essential, needed. It is not stopped. *nirbandhaḥ kṛṣṇa, anāsaktasya viṣayān yathārham upayuñjataḥ.* Don't be attached to the sense gratification. Just like eating, it is also a kind of sense gratification, to satisfy the tongue, satisfy the belly. But eating is also necessary if we want to maintain our body, and with the body you have to execute Kṛṣṇa consciousness. Without maintaining the body, or disturbing the body, we cannot.

So everything can be adjusted. That is Kṛṣṇa consciousness education. And we are trying to establish an ideal colony in New Vrindaban and other places. So I'm glad that in spite of all difficulties you are trying to... But do it nicely. Plain living, high thinking, that is required. It is not necessary that unnecessarily we increase objectives of sense gratification and be entangled. Minimize it and live peacefully, chant Hare Kṛṣṇa.

(Lecture on Śrīmad-Bhāgavatam 7.6.10,
New Vrindaban, June 26, 1976)

This verse is very significant for those desiring to elevate themselves to a higher level of Kṛṣṇa consciousness. When a person is initiated by a spiritual master, he changes his habits and does not eat undesirable eatables or engage in the eating of meat, the drinking of liquor, illicit sex or gambling. *Sāttvikā-āhāra*, foodstuffs in the mood of goodness, are described in the *Śāstras* as wheat, rice, vegetables, fruits, milk, sugar, and milk products. Simple food like rice, *dāl*, *capātīs*, vegetables, milk and sugar constitute a balanced diet, but sometimes it is found that an initiated person, in the name of *prasāda*, eats very luxurious foodstuffs. Due to his past sinful life he becomes attracted by Cupid and eats good food voraciously. It is clearly visible that when a neophyte in Kṛṣṇa consciousness eats too much, he falls down. Instead of being elevated to pure Kṛṣṇa consciousness, he becomes attracted by Cupid. The so-called *brahmacārī* becomes agitated by women, and the *vānaprastha* may again become captivated into having sex with his wife. Or he may begin to search out another wife.

(*Śrīmad-Bhāgavatam* 4.26.13, purport)

Yet they must take a lesson from the life of Bharata Mahārāja, to be very cautious and to see that not a single moment is wasted in frivolous talk, sleep or voracious eating. Eating is not prohibited, but if we eat voraciously we shall certainly sleep more than required. Sense gratification ensues, and we may be: degraded to a lower life form. In that way our spiritual progress may be checked at least for the time being.

(Śrīmad-Bhāgavatam 5.8.29, purport)

By overeating, an ordinary human being becomes prone to a disease called *amla-pitta*, which is a product of indigestion characterized by acidity of the stomach.

(Caitanya-caritāmṛta, Antya-līlā 10.19)

Fasting

Fasting effectively drives away disease. But your fasting should never impede your devotional service.

Regarding your fasting, if you are sick, then fasting is the best medicine. For disease and unwanted guests, if you do not give them food, they will go away.
(Letter to Revatīnandana Swami, January 16, 1975)

Disease is to be cured, is to be driven away. In Hindi they say, *jarā ar para okhane kha na baviya ar.* (?) Means "Unwanted guest and disease, you do not give him to eat, and he will go away." He will go away. So any disease, you starve for few days, two days, three days, it will go. And any unwanted guest, you don't supply him food. He will automatically go away. So disease should not be maintained. Disease should be cured.
(Lecture on Bhagavad-gita 7.2, London, March 10, 1975)

Hanṣadūta said that the preoccupation of many Western devotees seemed to be simply how to maintain their bodies. Adjusting to India was difficult, and many get sick. At the same time, he added, they do not control their eating habits, so they get into a cycle of over-eating and disease. "This is one of our biggest problems. Just as you say, when someone gets sick he should fast. I tell them, 'Stop eating. You'll get well immediately. If you have fever, don't eat. Take water, lemon. You'll be all right in a few days.' They have not realized how their own body is functioning, and they insist on eating. They get sicker and sicker, they complicate things. I've seen so many people get incredibly complicated digestive diseases. Then they can't work. They get jaundice, they get dysentery, amoebic dysentery, boils – all these things come from taking too much food. And then they want to change their diet. Although they change their diet, they eat so much of the changed diet that it also has no effect. And then they require money for medicine; I have spent so much money on medicine. Now I have stopped it. I tell them, 'First you fast for three days, and if you don't get better I'll give you some money for medicine.' But they are constantly running to this hospital, getting this pill and that pill. All these pills are useless. The real problem is they are just overeating. And of course when they overeat they want to sleep. Because India is hot. And when they sleep then they get dysentery. And when they get dysentery they can't engage. And in this way they run into a cycle which is very difficult to break.

"Only very few devotees are able to maintain themselves in India for any length of time. I see a nice strong man comes, and I look at him and

I see him eat, and I say, 'Within a week this man is going to be sick.' And sure enough, he's sick. He's lying down, he's got fever, he's got dysentery, he's going to the hospital. In this way we have so many people like that."

A wry smile appeared on Prabhupāda's face. "I have seen. Some of them eat so much I am surprised." He sat back and looked at his leaders. "So, how to manage this? It is very difficult."

(Transcendental Diary, Vol. 4, Chap. 5, October 4, 1976)

If one can fast, that is *tapasya*, Prabhupāda said, but it should not be artificial. Just like Raghunātha dāsa Gosvāmī. He was fasting, but he was not just fasting. People fast artificially and become weak and cannot work; that is not required. If you fast and at the same time you do not become weak, then that is recommended. And if after fasting you cannot do service, then what is the use of fasting?

Raghunātha Gosvāmī was fasting, but he was thrice taking bath and offering obeisances hundreds of times. His regular activities were not stopped, and he was taking every alternate day a little quantity of butter. That's all. It is not possible to imitate him. We have to work.

(Śrīla Prabhupāda Nectar, Nectar, Vol. 3, No. 13)

Foods and Herbs and Spices

Śrīla Prabhupāda's instructions about food, herbs, and spices.

Aloe Vera and Garlic

Surendra Saigal came in to Prabhupāda's room to find out what he wanted for breakfast. Prabhupāda mentioned apples and milk. Since Mr. Saigal had made some suggestions to Śrīla Prabhupāda for helping with his health, I asked him if he could get some *ghrita-kumari*, aloe vera. Arjuna and Tamopahā prabhu suggested it last week as a good remedy for high blood pressure and for cleaning the arteries. Mr. Saigal happily informed us that he had it growing in his garden. His wife takes it regularly, stuffed in *chapatis* or *parathas* (fried bread stuffed with potatoes or other vegetables) and finds it quite efficacious for relieving pains in her knees. Mr. Saigal though, suggested that garlic was the best for relieving high blood pressure.

Prabhupāda wrinkled his nose and grimaced slightly. "Garlic."

Mr. Saigal smiled at his reaction. "Garlic. You don't want it," and they laughed together.

"Garlic, onions, prohibited," Prabhupāda told him.

So it was settled that his wife would cook aloe vera *chapatis* for breakfast. Prabhupāda asked Gaurasundara prabhu if he knew of it, and he confirmed they had it in Hawaii. He added that it can be used externally for skin diseases, burns, and cuts.

As Mr. Saigal left the room to prepare for breakfast, Prabhupāda concluded, "Body is simply troublesome."

(Transcendental Diary, Vol. 5, Chap. 1, October 9, 1976)

Boysenberries

Once I gave Prabhupāda something with fresh boysenberries. He said, "Oh, this is very good. What is this?" I said, "That's called boysenberries. It's a cross between a couple of different kinds of berries by a man named Boysen." Prabhupāda said, "It is very good. Poison berry?" I said, "No, sir, boysenberry." He laughed; he was joking. So I told the devotees that story. I was one of Prabhupāda's lighthearted joking moods. Sometimes late, boysenberries were in the kitchen, and one of the *matajis* (ladies) said, "You can't offer those, they're poisonous. Prabhupāda said they're poisonous." I told Prabhupāda, "You joked with me about boysenberries and poison berries, and now the story is out that boysenberries are poisonous." He laughed and said, "Everyone is saying, "Prabhupāda has said this, and Prabhupāda has said that, but I've never said. Believe what you read in my books and what you hear me speak, and take everything else with a grain of salt."

(Interview with Nanda Kumar Dāsa)

Castor Seeds

Produce oil from castor seeds and stock the oil sufficiently. It can be used in so many ways—for burning, grease, cooking, and as a purgative to cure all diseases.

(Letter to Nityānanda Dāsa, March 16, 1977)

Chili

He noticed a small chili bush at the side of the temple so as he took his breakfast this morning he sent me out to pick a few. They were very little and I did not think they would be very strong. Prabhupāda took but a small bite of one and left it at the side of his plate. Several minutes later he raised his eyebrows and said, "It is very hot!" Concerned that it might be burning his mouth I asked if it was too hot, but he simply smiled. "No, chili *means* hot."

(Transcendental Diary, Vol. 2, Chap. 4, May 8, 1976)

Chickpeas

Prabhupāda once asked about the health of the New Vrindaban community's horse. A disciple said the horse was sick. Prabhupāda told the devotee to feed the horse chickpeas. He said chickpeas are very good for horses and make them strong.

(Conversation, London, August 26, 1973)

Once I was carrying Prabhupāda's plate through the *prasādam* room when I heard someone say, "In New York Prabhupāda told us that you could only serve seven chickpeas."
Somebody else said, "No, no, it's eleven.
I heard it in Los Angeles."
Somebody else said, "No, it's twenty-one.
Prabhupāda told us that."
I went into Prabhupāda's room and gave him his plate and said, "Śrīla Prabhupāda, there's a controversy about how many chickpeas we can eat. Some say seven, some say eleven, some say twenty-one."

He gave the same answer. He said, "Everyone is quoting this and that and this and that. Believe what you hear from me directly and what you hear in my books. And as far as chickpeas are concerned, eat as many as you can digest."

(Interview with Nanda Kumar Dāsa)

Iron Pills

I am glad to learn that Jadurāṇī is feeling a little better and I hope you will take proper care of the girl. I understand that Govinda dāsī has recommended Jadurāṇī to take iron pills and almost all the girls here are taking them. It is compensating for the deficiency due to their past habit of meat taking. This is a good recommendation and I hope Jadurāṇī is trying to follow it. Here it is understood that Nandarāṇī, Śyāmā dāsī and others are feeling better from taking iron medicine."

(Letter to Satsvarūpa Dāsa, November 18, 1968)

Nima (Neem)

Those leaves are *nima* leaves. Keep them and when I come there I shall make a preparation of toothpaste. *Nima* tree is very antiseptic.

(Letter to Brahmānanda, March 21, 1968)

Ḍākinī and Śāṅkhinī are two companions of Lord Śiva and his wife who are supposed to be extremely inauspicious, having been born of ghostly life. It is believed that such inauspicious living creatures cannot go near a *nima* tree. At least medically it is accepted that *nima* wood is extremely antiseptic, and formerly it was customary to have a *nima* tree in front of one's house. On very large roads in India, especially in Uttar Pradesh, there are hundreds and thousands of *nima* trees. *Nima* wood is so antiseptic that the Āyurvedic science uses it to cure leprosy. Medical scientists have extracted the active principle of the *nima* tree, which is called margosic acid. *Nima* is used for many purposes, especially to brush the teeth. In Indian villages ninety percent of the people use *nima* twigs for this purpose. Because of all the antiseptic effects of the *nima* tree and because Lord Caitanya was born beneath a *nima* tree, Sītā Ṭhākurāṇī gave the Lord the name Nimāi.

(Caitanya-caritāmṛta, Ādi-līlā 13.117, purport)

Ghee

You inquire whether you can make cheese? Why cheese? Make sufficient ghee. If you can send ghee to India that would be nice service as there is scarcely any ghee there. Cheese is not good. We should produce ghee so all our centers can have enough ghee.

(Letter to Kīrtanānanda Dāsa, January 7, 1974)

Mangoes

"In Miami there are so many mangoes and coconuts. I am enjoying the dobs from Florida. The orange ones especially are very nice. I am taking one each day. From the green mangoes you can make pickles. Cut them into pieces with skin intact, and sprinkle with salt and turmeric. Dry them well in the sunshine and put into mustard oil. They will keep for years and you can enjoy with eating. They are nice and soft and good for digestion. If no vegetable is available, you can eat them with *purīs*, similarly with pickled chilies. When mango pickles and chili pickles are combined, it is very tasteful. The Miami temple sounds to be very nice with bathing place and peacocks, just like Vṛndāvana. Kṛṣṇa will supply you everything, don't worry. Just work sincerely."

(Letter to Balavanta Dasa, July 8, 1976)

Milk for Expecting Mothers

Prabhupāda was always very concerned that his devotees maintain their health. One time he expressed this concern to one of his spiritual daughters who was pregnant, and he gave her advice about health.

When Prabhupāda was in Philadelphia. Sarveśvarī Dāsī would cook for him. Once, when she went into Prabhupāda's room to remove his plate, she noticed that there was a full cup of milk left. Prabhupāda told her she should drink it. He said she should drink as much as possible while she was pregnant and nursing and in this way her baby would be very happy, healthy and peaceful. Sarveśvarī Dāsī said she would drink the milk and she took his plate away.

As Sarveśvarī carried Prabhupāda's plate down the stairs, Brahmānanda passed her and spotted the milk. Give me that milk! he said. But Sarveśvarī said she couldn't because Prabhupāda had told her to drink it. Brahmānanda then conceded that she needed it more than he.

(Śrīla Prabhupāda Nectar, Vol. 5, No. 29)

Milk is Nectar

Milk is compared to nectar, which one can drink to become immortal. Of course, simply drinking milk will not make one immortal, but it can increase the duration of one's life. In modern civilization, men do not think milk to be important, and therefore they do not live very long. Although in this age men can live up to one hundred years, their duration of life is reduced because they do not drink large quantities of milk. This is a sign of Kali-yuga.

In Kali-yuga, instead of drinking milk, people prefer to slaughter an animal and eat its flesh. The Supreme Personality of Godhead, in His instructions of *Bhagavad-gītā*, advises *go-rakṣya*, which means cow protection. The cow should be protected, milk should be drawn from the cows, and this milk should be prepared in various ways.

One should take ample milk, and thus one can prolong one's life, develop his brain, execute devotional service, and ultimately attain the favor of the Supreme Personality of Godhead. As it is essential to get food grains and water by digging the earth, it is also essential to give protection to the cows and take nectarean milk from their milk bags...

The so-called *vaiśyas* — the industrialists or businessmen — are involved in big, big industrial enterprises, but they are not interested in food grains and milk. However, as indicated here, by digging for water, even in the desert, we can produce food grains; when we produce food grains and vegetables, we can give protection to the cows; while giving protection to the cows, we can draw from them abundant quantities of milk; and by getting enough milk and combining it with food grains and vegetables, we can prepare hundreds of nectarean foods. We can happily eat this food and thus avoid industrial enterprises and joblessness.

(Śrīmad-Bhāgavatam 8.6.12, purport)

"*Go-rakṣya*, the point is that cow's milk is very important," Prabhupāda replied. "Therefore specifically mentioned *go-rakṣya*. Kṛṣṇa does not say that don't eat meat. It is not clearly said that meat-eating is forbidden. But meat-eating is tamasic. But He's speaking of *go-rakṣya* for our special material benefit, that if we protect the cows, we can have the facility of drinking milk, which will help us in keeping our health in order and developing very nice brain tissues to understand spiritual subject matter.

Meat-eaters, they're all dull. They cannot understand finer philosophy of life. Meat-eating, not good. But the *Śūdras*, and less than *Śūdras*, they eat. But for them there's lower animals, not cow."

(Transcendental Diary, Vol. 2, Chap. 4, May 30, 1976)

Milk and Halavā

Regarding your need for a warm beverage to drink while you are working, milk is the best. Take hot milk with a little sugar, stir it very nicely, and drink it when it is warm sufficiently, tolerable by you, and with bubbles on the surface. That is the best hot beverage available in the world. You can also prepare some *halevāh*. That is also very nice for a cold country. Add to it some raisins, almonds, etc.

(Letter to Śivānanda Dāsa, May 4, 1969)

Milk and Salt

Milk and salt should never be mixed. It is improper and will cause leprosy. But salt can be mixed with yogurt.

(Letter to Aniruddha Dāsa, April 9, 1968)

Yogurt

Sudāmā also rode with us, holding several bottles of a liquid milk culture called keifer. He told Prabhupāda that the keifer was very good for the devotees' health, but Śrīla Prabhupāda said he didn't want any. It was better he said, to use fresh boiled milk, or to make your own yogurt.

(Life with the Perfect Master, Chap. 2)

Dried – Banana Chips

If you take green bananas, peel them and put them out in the sun to dry for one, two, three days – til it is dry – then these may be sent to me, especially when I go to Europe. This is a very good tonic for liver, and I am now having these unripened bananas daily in Los Angeles.

(Letter to Govinda Dāsī, August 17, 1969)

Śrīmati Jayaśrī Dāsī has sent me some dried banana chips and they are very nice for my Ekādaśī food. Is it possible to send us in large quantity this foodstuff? If not, please try to send me at least one small packet like that every fortnight. It is very nice. The mango pulp, a sample of which was also sent to me, I don't think it has come out very nice, so there is no need of sending it.

(Letter to Gaurasundara Dāsa, November 20, 1969)

Rice, Dāl, and Chapattis, etc.

My first concern is that you are not eating well. It is a case of anxiety. Please don't eat *dāl* & spices. Simply boiled vegetables, rice & a few *chapattis*. Take butter separately and eat only as much as you may require for taste. Drink milk twice, morning & evening. Use some digestive pill after each principle meal. I think soda-mint tablets will help. Be careful about your health first. This information is not only for you but for all my noble sons. I am an old man. I may live or die it does not matter. But you must live for long time to push on this Kṛṣṇa consciousness movement.

(Letter to Rāyarāma Dāsa, December 21, 1967)

I am anxious to know how you are eating, whether you have got the facilities for cooking nice *prasādam*. Japanese rice is very cheap, so if you take nice rice, *dāl*, *capātīs*, vegetable and little milk, that will keep your health nice.

(Letter to Bali Mardana Dāsa and Sudāmā Dāsa, October 3, 1969)

Puffed Rice

Prabhupāda: My mother used to make puffed rice at home. So there is special rice available for making puffed rice.

Either you can prepare at home or you can purchase in the market, special rice. So she was preparing nice puffed rice, very, very nice. In a sand pot. My mother was always engaged in making some food preparation. Some pickled, some chutney, and this puffed rice, or something else, something else, something else. Besides cooking for the family, she was being assisted by my sisters. Always palatable foodstuff. So many guests were there, and

if son-in-law would come, they would specially prepare food for him. To receive guests, give them nice food to eat, prepare nice food for the family, this is the Indian pleasure. They are not very much, nowadays, for upkeep of the home, very...That, in their own way, they keep it very nicely. Every utensils, very cleansed, they are kept ready for use, some cloth. If you go in a poor man's home, but you'll find everything very neat and clean. Ask these *gṛhasthas* to keep their home very neat and clean. Are they keeping?
Bhagavān: Yes.
Prabhupāda: What is the general program for eating?
Bhagavān: For eating? Every morning everyone has a nice glass of yogurt, chickpeas and apple, orange and banana.
Prabhupāda: Chickpeas fried?
Bhagavān: Boiled, chick peas. And people, orange and banana. And in the afternoon they have rice, *dāl*, *chapati*, and salad, and in a little bread.
Prabhupāda: That's nice.

(Conversation, New Mayapur, August 3, 1976)

At about 8:30 p.m. Prabhupāda was talking with Bhagavān in his room, once again discussing the important role of food and its preparation in self-sufficient living. He described how to make puffed rice by heating sand in one container and then dumping it on top of the grains in another pot. "It will puff-puff-puff-puff-puff-puff, they'll be finished." By straining it all through a mesh you end up with the puffed-up grains, which he said was "very good food."

When I told him the devotees make popcorn he said that was "not very digestive;" puffed rice however, is very light. "In the morning you can give them this puffed grains, then fruits and milk – very good breakfast. I mean to say, all self-dependent. Yes, we should save time, as much for this purpose, for chanting, discussing *grantha* (scripture). Not for any personal so-called comforts. We can sit down anywhere on the grass here, and whatever available we make our food. This is the idea. Life will be sublime.

(Transcendental Diary, Vol. 3, Chap. 5, August 3, 1976)

Spices

Prabhupāda is attempting to treat his disease by adjusting the spicing in his diet. In the morning he instructed Pālikā to soak black pepper and cumin seed and then grind them into a paste. He had her do the same with turmeric. She cooked his lunch using this spicing, carefully mixing the paste with the required amount of water and adding it to his lunch preparations. Then this evening he called her in and had her make two *parathas* and a potato and eggplant *subji.* We were delighted to see him eat and he told us that the spicing had given him a good appetite.

(Transcendental Diary, Vol. 4, Chap. 2, August 15, 1976)

Prabhupāda's main health program was his diet, but even in that he was not very strict. An Indian cook named Shantilal was present in Bhuvaneśvara, and he used a lot of spices and ghee in cooking for Gargamuni Swami and his men. Sometimes Prabhupāda would ask for some of what Shantilal had cooked, and this greatly disturbed Prabhupāda's servants and cooks, although they could do nothing about it. Gargamuni had also been ill recently, and when Prabhupāda first saw him with his cook Shantilal, he had said, "I thought you were sick."

"Yes," Gargamuni had replied, "but still I have to eat. Śrīla Prabhupāda, you are eating very simply. You are not eating spiced food?"

"Sometimes I also have to have spices," Prabhupāda replied. "Otherwise there is no taste. And without that taste, what is the use of life?" Then in a joking spirit Prabhupāda and Gargamuni Swami commiserated, saying they were not going to stop eating tasty *prasādam.*

"We'd rather die," laughed Gargamuni Swami, and Prabhupāda also laughed.

(Śrīla Prabhupāda–līlāmṛta Chap. 51)

Watermelon

Along with a flower garland and fresh sandalwood paste (cooling paste made from the pulp of sandwood) I have also been offering Prabhupāda watermelon every afternoon after his post-lunch nap. The melons are so large that I only use a portion and save the rest in the refrigerator for later use. Śrīla Prabhupāda happened to notice it and told me to stop, declaring, "Cut fruit must be distributed immediately."

(Transcendental Diary, Vol. 4, Chap. 2, August 15, 1976)

Water

Due to weakness and ill health, Prabhupāda is taking some *dahlia*, cracked wheat, with his milk in the evening. It helps with a better bowel movement, and he has been feeling some benefit from it the last couple of days. Another thing that has helped his digestion is some water from Bhubaneswar in Orissa, from the Bindu Sarovar lake. A Calcutta devotee, Debu, brought a 20-gallon container of it across India on the train because he had heard that it has curative and health-giving properties. Prabhupāda has been drinking it regularly and says he is benefiting from it.

(Transcendental Diary, Vol. 5, Chap. 3, November 5, 1976)

Once after silently demonstrating his technique of drinking water, Prabhupāda said to a boy who was present, "You cannot do that." One reason for drinking in that manner was cleanliness; one's lip or mouth doesn't touch the edge of the drinking vessel. Prabhupāda would pour the water down, swallowing, and then tilting the chalice upright, stop the flow of water without spilling a drop.

In India, the water would be kept cool in big clay jugs. In the West, water was served with ice sometimes. Once when Prabhupāda asked for water, his servant asked, "Do you want cold water?" Prabhupāda replied, "Water means cold water."

And water must be covered. In India, to leave a clay jug of water uncovered is, he said, "signing your death warrant." In the West, the pitcher also should be covered.

He could appreciate different tastes of water. We would make efforts to get him the best water from special sources, like Bhagatiji's well in Vṛndāvana.

He would drink quite a bit of water for health and digestion. He would make comments about it as we sat with him in his room watching him drink water. But don't draw his water from a bathroom! Pradyumna dāsa asked how it is actually different if the water comes from the bathroom, provided one doesn't know where the water comes from. Prabhupāda replied that it would affect the mind, even if you didn't know where the water came from, because the bathroom is a contaminated place.

Only a disciple could know how sweet it was to talk about these apparently mundane things. To confer with Prabhupāda about his needs or to talk about water was relief from greater problems. One thought, "Let me stay here and supply Prabhupāda water so he can preach and write books; nothing else is as important as his water, his health, his daily *Bhāgavatam* work, his being pleased. Nothing is as nice to see as his drinking, as the water falls from the cup to his mouth."

(Śrīla Prabhupāda Nectar Nectar, Vol. 1, No. 41)

Undesirable Food

To live within this material world one must face many dangers, as described herein. For example, undesirable food possesses a danger to health, and therefore one must give up such food, the Dhanvantari incarnation can protect in this regard. Since Lord Viṣṇu is the Supersoul of all living entities, if he likes He can save us from *adhibhautika* disturbances, disturbances from other living entities. Lord Balarāma is the Śeṣa incarnation, and therefore He can save us from angry serpents or envious persons, who are always ready to attack.

(Śrīmad-Bhāgavatam 6.8.18, purport)

Avoid Food Purchased in the Market

Your second question, ice cream purchased from the market may not be offered. Because such ice cream contains sometimes undesirable things, which we should not offer. We must offer to Kṛṣṇa only first class prepared foodstuff, especially made at home. We shall try to avoid as far as possible goods purchased from the market and offer to Kṛṣṇa.

(Letter to Śyāmā Dāsī, October 21, 1968)

Chocolate and Frozen Vegetables

Just a further point about Śrīla Prabhupāda's having accepted chocolate in the early days of his preaching in the West but then in 1976 telling us that because it is made from cacao it cannot be taken. There is a parallel in his view of frozen food.

In Vṛndāvana on November 3, 1976 myself and Haṁsadūta were

having a chat with His Divine Grace and the subject of frozen food came up:

Haṁsadūta Swami has been several times to Moscow to visit with Ananta Santi prabhu, Prabhupāda's only Russian disciple, and he and Prabhupāda shared some observations and realizations about the poor quality of life there. Ananta Santi's entire family lives in a couple of rooms half the size of Śrīla Prabhupāda's *darśana* room, taxi drivers beg money from their clients and the only vegetables available are frozen.

Prabhupāda screwed his face a little in disgust. That is also nasty. Frozen means nasty. I never take frozen. In the beginning I thought, 'Oh, it is very nice, you can get fresh vegetable.' But they are not at all fresh. All rotten. Rather the same vegetable, as we have got in Indian practice, we dry it and keep it. That is tasteful. The point is that initially, when he first came across frozen food he thought it was nice. But later on he declared it 'nasty' and tamasic (in the mode of ignorance):

As he lay in the half light, I mentioned that I had heard some of the temples were using frozen foods for their Deity offerings. Prabhupāda shook his head and gave a sour look. Tamasic food, tamasic activities! It is going on simply by Kṛṣṇa's mercy!

Similarly, Śrīla Prabhupāda may have accepted chocolate at one point, but later, he rejected it. So there is no contradiction in the evidences presented from Yamunā, Indradyumna Swami, etc., and myself. The last instruction is the one we follow.

(Letter from Hari Śauri Dāsa, August 2, 1976)

Haṁsadūta: No, he said, I was able to get frozen vegetables from the south of Russia. They freeze it and then they sell it, he said, but it is very expensive, very costly. He was getting frozen.
Prabhupāda: That is also nasty. Frozen means nasty. I never take frozen. In the beginning I thought, Oh, it is very nice, you can get fresh vegetable. But they are not at all fresh.
Haṁsadūta: No.
Prabhupāda: All rotten, rather the same vegetable, as we have got in India practice, we dry it and keep it. That is tasteful. In season time — suppose this season there is huge quantity of vegetable — so here the system is they cut into pieces during the season and dry it in the sun and

keep it. And during out of season it is soaked in water, it revives the old taste, and then you can cook.

Devotee: Tastes as though it is different. The fresh vegetable the taste is very good.

Prabhupāda: Fresh vegetable must be, but still there is some taste. But this frozen it has no taste.

(Conversation, Vrindavan, November 3, 1976)

Prabhupāda: So you will never discover the cure, and he will never come out. Now somebody was saying that this freezing, the body within, they decompose. The parts of the body are separate. That is...As we have... You take the frozen vegetable. It is tasteless. It is decomposed.

(Morning Walk, Los Angeles, July 24, 1975)

For weeks Śrīla Prabhupāda had been taking a commercially prepared food supplement, Complain, but now he refused it. What is the use of artificial food, he said, when there is natural? You Westerners like the taste of canned, frozen, preserved, rotten food. You eat and then keep the leftovers for seven months, and this you like.

(Śrīla Prabhupāda–līlāmṛta 53: Kṛṣṇa's Great Soldier)

Prabhupāda turned to Rāma dāsa. "This is very nice. Are the peas fresh?" Rāma dāsa, embarrassed, explained that they were frozen. Prabhupāda gave Rāma dāsa an intense look. "Frozen peas should never be offered to Kṛṣṇa."

(Great Transcendental Adventure Chap. 13)

Don't Eat Too Much Sweet

Those who have studied...The ants are very much fond of being intoxicated. Therefore, they find out sweet, sugar. Sweet is intoxication. Perhaps you know, all. The liquor is made from sugar. Sugar is fermented with acid, sulphuric acid, and then it is distilled. That is liquor. Therefore too much sweet eating is prohibited.

(Lecture on Bhagavad-gītā 2.19-20, London, August 25, 1973)

No Soybeans

Prabhupāda once asked Nandarāṇī dāsī if her children ate *dāl* and *chapattis* every day. At that time the children were ages one and two. Nandarāṇī said yes, and Prabhupāda approved. He said that if children ate *dāl* and *chapattis* from the time they were young, they would always be healthy. He said the *dāl* should be very hot that she should soak the *chapatti* until it was very soft, and then children could eat it. He said she could mix rice in the *dāl* as well. Prabhupāda said that *urad dāl* is the best, then mung, then lentils, but that soybeans are not needed.

(Śrīla Prabhupāda Nectar Vol. 5, No. 29)

Cleanliness

The main work of the GBC is to train the devotees in the standards of internal and external cleanliness.

So you must live up to the rules and regulations of brahminical life. First and foremost is cleanliness. In your country they have so many filthy habits. For example, they don't wash after eating. A *brāhmaṇa* does not do like that. If he did so in India, he would be highly criticized. So even if you eat a little, still you must wash immediately. And the place that you eat at must be washed off immediately also.

(Letter to Lakṣmī Nārāyaṇa Dāsa, Los Angeles, July 8, 1971)

We have got such a nice process that even from the base *Śūdras* we can create *brāhmaṇas* of highest caliber. All the presidents of our centers should see that all the members are strictly observing the brahminical standards, such as rising early, cleansing at least twice daily, reading profusely, and attending *ārati*, like that. You begin immediately this process. That is the main work of GBC. Sometimes we see that even they do not wash hands after eating. Even after drinking water we should wash hands. That is *Śuci*. *Śuci* means purest.

(Letter to Rūpānuga Dāsa, Tokyo, May 3, 1972)

One should also be clean, within and without. To be outwardly clean, one should regularly bathe with soap and oil, and to be inwardly clean one should always be absorbed in thoughts of Kṛṣṇa.

(Caitanya-caritāmṛta, Madhya-Līlā 23.109, purport)

There was only one letter to reply to today, from Kīrtanānanda Swami, who reported his reason for not being able to attend the festival. The West Virginia state health authorities had placed a quarantine order on New Vrindaban because some devotees had become sick with jaundice. Kīrtanānanda Mahārāja said that some inimical state authorities overreacted to the situation. Now he thinks their community will be obliged to accept some regulation by the state authorities. His mood has been to keep things as simple as possible, but, as he admitted, "either due to their lack of vision, or our lack of expertise, simplicity has been taken for dirtiness."

In his reply, Prabhupāda told him if it is necessary to make alterations he may do so. Yet, he clearly stated his opinion of the modern so-called sanitary arrangements in the West. "If the water supply is sufficient, there is no question of insanitation. Disease comes when there are dirty conditions...Concerning the [existing] outhouses, if they are not approved then you can have a septic tank, or pass stool in the open field. I was doing that. I never liked to go to the nonsense toilet so I was going in the field."

(Transcendental Diary, Vol. 1, Chap. 10, March 23, 1976)

Today was Ekādaśī, and Śrīla Prabhupāda took his morning walk along the Gaṅgā. Hundreds of pilgrims were taking a dawn bath there, having come for the Gaṅgā-Sāgara-*melā*. Prabhupāda explained that *sagara* is the sea, so the *melā* is a spiritual gathering on an island in the Gaṅgā's estuary.

Evidently eager pilgrims had traveled from as far away as Rajasthan in the northwest. They camped along the banks of Mother Gaṅgā, washing their few possessions, as well as themselves, in the holy waters, unmindful of the boats and other river traffic passing by. They sat contentedly on the pathways cooking breakfast and drying out their clothing.

Noting the shining *loṭā* (water pot) one man carried, Prabhupāda remarked that if even the *loṭā* is so clean, we can understand how clean he must personally be.

(Transcendental Diary, Vol. 1, Chap. 8, January 13, 1976)

Exercise

Taking walks and bathing in the sea (whenever possible) will help you keep your body fit for devotional service.

Too Much Not Necessary

After Nālinī-kānta read Prahlāda Māharaja's analysis of the one hundred years of human life, how it becomes wasted by material activities like sporting and economic endeavor, Prabhupāda invited his guests, "Now discuss on this point. If anyone has objection. Yes, Dr. Wolf."

"Do not some physical means come into the keeping the body strong, healthy, so that devotion is possible at all? Because to produce sick people, of course, is not in the Lord's spirit either, I think."

"No. Our aim is not to create sick people," Prabhupāda told him. "That is not our aim."

"Swimming, walking, is still important I think."

"No, we do not say. Neither."

"I miss it in the Movement," Dr. Wolf told him. "I think it should not be made a sport, but it should be made, perhaps, a physical 'must,' under control."

Although Prabhupāda affirmed that good health was necessary, he didn't agree that it required some special regimen or arrangement. "No, if you eat more, then you require more exercise to digest unnecessary loading; but if you eat simply, just to keep our body and soul together, you don't require exercise. Little movement is going on, we are walking. But not this severe type of exercise as surfers and fighting with the sea waves for four hours, five hours, ten hours."

(Transcendental Diary, Vol. 2, Chap. 5, June 10, 1976)

Swimming and Bathing in the Ocean

The next morning, from the porch, Śrīla Prabhupāda was watching the devotees swimming in the Bay of Bengal. Calling Hari-śauri over, he said he would like to bathe in the ocean and asked him what he thought about it. Hari-śauri and the other devotees present all thought it was a good idea. Sea water was supposed to be very good for health, they said. Prabhupāda said he would try it and after taking his morning massage walked down to the seashore, wearing his *gamchā* and carrying a towel. The ocean shore was about a hundred yards from the hotel, and by the time Prabhupāda reached the water, all the devotees were running after him in their *gamchās*.

Some of the devotees were already in the ocean, and when Prabhupāda reached the water's edge, they all gathered around him. As the waves glided in and swirled around Prabhupāda's feet, Hari-śauri scooped palmfuls of water and began to bathe Prabhupāda's body-his arms, chest, and head-washing away the mustard seed oil he had applied during the massage. Soon other devotees began reverently splashing handfuls of water onto Prabhupāda's body. Standing almost up to his knees in water, the bright sunshine illuminating his golden-hued body, Prabhupāda laughed as the devotees joined in.

The devotees realized that this pastime was just like an *abhiṣeka*, or bathing of the Deity, and when Guru-kṛpā Swami began to sing the prayers for bathing the Deity – *cintāmaṇi-prakara-sadmasu* – the other devotees joined in, singing and taking part in the *abhiṣeka* (sacred bath of the Deities) by the sea. Śrīla Prabhupāda enjoyed it, sometimes putting his head forward to indicate that he wanted water poured on his head, then closing his eyes as the devotees poured the water. When Prabhupāda lost his balance for a moment, Hari-śauri grabbed him. Prabhupāda's feet had been sinking into the sand, and when he held one foot out it was muddy. As he wriggled his toes, a devotee poured water on the foot, washing it clean. Prabhupāda then bent over, put ocean water in his mouth, and spat it out. Only Guru-kṛpā Swami was quick enough to catch some of the water and drink it.

As Prabhupāda allowed the devotees to participate in bathing and gently massaging him, the devotees were carried away by ecstatic feelings. After about ten minutes, Prabhupāda came out of the water, changed his clothes, and walked back to the hotel, where two devotees escorted him to a comfortable chair, sat him down, and carried him up to his room for his afternoon rest.

(**Śrīla Prabhupāda**–*līlāmṛta Chap. 51)*)

Wake Up Early and Morning Walks

When Śrīla Prabhupāda was having what appeared to be a heart attack, doctor came who recommended that he take a daily

morning walk. When Śrīla Prabhupāda recovered from his illness, he began to take daily walks.

It was getting worse—total weakness and everything. I couldn't get a doctor, because it was Memorial Day and everything was closed. I even called my family doctor, but he wasn't in. Everyone had gone on vacation, because on Memorial Day everyone leaves the city. I couldn't get anyone. I was calling hospitals, doctors – trying this and that. But I couldn't get anyone. Finally I got a doctor by calling an emergency number for the New York City medical department. The doctor came. He was an old geezer with a real loud voice. When he saw Swamiji he said, "I think the old man is praying too much. I think he should get some exercise. He should go out for a walk in the morning."

(Śrīla Prabhupāda–*līlāmṛta Chap.25*)

In our childhood with my father I used to walk 10 miles to save a ticket of 5 paise (Indian coin) on the tram car. So we are trained up in that way. Of course it was a very pleasant morning walk.

(Letter to Tamāla Kṛṣṇa Dāsa, London, September 1, 1971)

Early in the morning at half past seven. If he walks early in the morning, all his disease will be cured. That he will not do. After all, everyone can do after performing *maṅgala-ārātrika*, take a morning walk.

(Morning Walk, Hyderabad, April, 23, 1974)

Prabhupāda: We have got activities day and night, but because the body is there, we have to eat, but we eat Kṛṣṇa *prasādam*. And naturally we go to sleep, to take some rest. Otherwise we are always engaged in Kṛṣṇa's business. We have no other business. So I go in the morning for little morning walk because the body, whole day if I sit down, it may be jammed.

(Conversation, Melbourne, April 23, 1976)

Prabhupāda: Oh yes. I was going to morning walk when there was snowfall. I was walking on snow.

(Conversation with Mr. Malhotra, *Poona, December 22, 1976)*

Yoga

Performing Yoga

Then Lord Kṛṣṇa says, *nātyaśnatas tu yogo 'sti.* Anyone who eats more than necessary, oh, he cannot perform yoga. *Na ati aśnatas tu yogo 'sti na ca ekāntam anaśnatah* [Bg. 6.16]. A person, I mean to say, willfully trying to keep himself in starvation, he cannot perform yoga. Neither the person who eats more than he requires, he also cannot perform yoga. The eating process should be moderate, only for keeping the body and soul together. Not for enjoyment of the tongue. So that is the real yogic process, that you cannot eat very palatable things. Because as soon as palatable things comes before us, naturally if I take one, I must take two, three, four. You see? So so far yogis are concerned, they cannot take any palatable desirable things. They have to simply take only the necessities. Some of the yogis, I have seen, there was one yogi in Calcutta...Of course, in a temple, in a sanctified place. He was taking once only a little quantity of rice boiled with water, at three o'clock in the afternoon he was taking. That was his food and nothing more. Nothing more.

(Lecture on Bhagavad-gītā 6.11–21, New York, September 7, 1966)

Sleep, Dreaming, Eating, and Yoga

So nātyaśnatas tu yogo 'sti na caikāntam anaśnataḥ na cāti svapna-śīlasya. If anyone dreams very much, he cannot also execute. Now, here Śrī Kṛṣṇa does not say that there is dreamless sleep. Dreamless sleep cannot be possible. It is not possible. If somebody says, dreamless sleep, it is also another lunacy. No. Dream there must be, more or less. As soon as you go asleep, oh, dream there must be. That may be good dream, bad dream, or for long time or for little time. But dream there must be. Now, Kṛṣṇa says that *na cāti svapna-śīlasya.* That means "One who dreams very much while sleeping, he cannot execute yoga." *Na jāgrato naiva cārjuna.* And one who cannot sleep at night...I have got a young friend, he cannot sleep. So for him, it is not yoga...yoga process is not possible. He may note down here. So sleep also required. You cannot remain without sleeping. That is also required. That means somehow or other, you should keep your body fit. You should not eat more, you sleeping.

That is also required. That means somehow or other, you should keep your body fit. You should not eat more, you shall not voluntarily starve, you should not be voluntarily awake, and neither, and if you keep yourself peaceful, then you'll not sleep...you'll not dream also. When the bile is very much agitated, then we see so many dreams due to the air which is coming out of agitated bile. And if you keep yourself peaceful, cool mind, cool head, cool, I mean to say, stomach, then there will, there will be ordinary sleep.

(Lecture on Bhagavad-gītā 6.11–21, New York, September 7, 1966)

Keep the Body Straight While Chanting

The Hare Kṛṣṇa *mahā-mantra*, however, may be chanted at any place and any time, and this will bring results very quickly. Yet even while chanting the Hare Kṛṣṇa mantra one may observe regulative principles. Thus while sitting and chanting one may keep his body straight, and this will help one in the chanting process; otherwise one may feel sleepy.

(Śrīmad-Bhāgavatam 7.15.31, purport)

Haṭha Yoga

Regarding other yoga exercises, if you take Kṛṣṇa *prasāda* you shall keep your body automatically fit for working, so there is no need of extra exercises which are required by persons who may eat more than what is required. So for prosecuting Kṛṣṇa consciousness one should not eat more than what is needed. One should not endeavor beyond his capacity. One should not talk unnecessarily. One should not stick with some extra regulative principles, nor should one associate with persons who are not in Kṛṣṇa consciousness. One should not be too much greedy. What one should do is chant the holy name of the Lord with faith, enthusiasm and firm conviction on the statement of Lord Caitanya that simply by chanting the *mahā-mantra* one can be gradually elevated to the highest platform of spiritual perfection. Also what is important is to follow the four regulative principles of avoiding illicit sexual connections, meat-eating, intoxication and gambling. I am sure that Rūpānuga will ably guide you in these matters.

(Letter to Kanupriya Dāsa, January 15, 1969)

Anyway I know the people of Tehran they like haṭha yoga very much. I understand Parivrājakācārya Swami is teaching a course combining both haṭha and bhakti yoga to attract the people. This is a very good idea. Somehow or other inject the bhakti yoga. That will save them from the degradations of sense gratification.

(Letter to Atreya Ṛṣi Dāsa, Bombay, Decemeber 4, 1974)

In Ayurveda, disease are said to originate in the improper digestion of which one cause may be that the airs of life (*vata*) are not circulating properly in the body.

Diseases of the body take place due to derangement of air within the earthly body of the living beings. Mental diseases result from special derangement of the air within the body, and as such, yogic exercise is especially beneficial to keep the air in order so that diseases of the body become almost nil by such exercises. When they are properly done the duration of life also increases, and one can have control over death also by such practices. A perfect yogi can have command over death and quit the body at the right moment, when he is competent to transfer himself to a suitable planet. The *bhakti-yogi*, however, surpasses all the yogis because, by dint of his devotional service, he is promoted to the region beyond the material sky and is placed in one of the planets in the spiritual sky by the supreme will of the Lord, the controller of everything.

(Śrīmad-Bhāgavatam 2.5.26–29, puport)

By good behavior and freedom from envy one should counteract sufferings due to other living entities, by meditation in trance one should counteract sufferings due to providence, and by practicing *haṭha-yoga, prāṇāyāma* [breath control to subdue the mind] and so forth one should counteract sufferings due to the body and mind. Similarly, by developing the mode of goodness, especially in regard to eating, one should conquer sleep.

(Śrīmad-Bhāgavatam 7.15.24)

By practice, one should avoid eating in such a way that other living entities will be disturbed and suffer. Since I suffer when pinched or killed by others, I should not attempt to pinch or kill any other living entity. People do not know that because of killing innocent animals they themselves will have to suffer severe reactions from material nature. Any country where people indulge in unnecessary killing of animals will have to suffer from wars and pestilence imposed by material nature. Comparing one's own suffering to the suffering of others, therefore, one should be kind to all living entities. One cannot avoid the sufferings inflicted by providence, and therefore when suffering comes one should fully absorb oneself in chanting the Hare Kṛṣṇa mantra. One can avoid sufferings from the body and mind by practicing mystic *haṭha-yoga.*

(Śrīmad-Bhāgavatam 7.15.24, purport)

Tamāla Kṛṣṇa: Parivrājakācārya Swami.
Prabhupāda: Very nice. Good combination.
Tamāla Kṛṣṇa: He's been there now, Parivrājakācārya Swami, he's been there now for, I think, two or three years now. He's worked pretty faithfully there. He tricks them. In the guise of teaching a little *haṭha-yoga*, then he teaches bhakti.
Prabhupāda: That is preaching.

(Conversation, Vṛndāvana, October 9, 1977)

While walking to a meadow, they came upon a man standing on his head.
"Is this our man?" Prabhupāda asked.
The devotees laughed and replied, "No, yoga."
"He wants to be immortal," said Rāmeśvara.
"No," said Prabhupāda. "This keeps them healthy."
Tamāla Kṛṣṇa: "It's good for the body?"
Prabhupāda: "Yes, *Śīrṣāsana* it is called, sitting on the head. *Śīrṣāsana, padmāsana, yogāsana*-there are so many *āsanas* [yogic postures]."
Tamāla Kṛṣṇa: "We don't practice those."
"Yes, we have no time from sleeping," said Prabhupāda sarcastically. The devotees laughed at his cutting remark. "Otherwise," Prabhupāda continued, this is not bad. This is not bad. It keeps good health, this *yoga-āsana.*

(Śrīla Prabhupāda Lilamrita Chap. 47)

Also, one of the things that I had to give up when I moved in the temple was hatha-yoga. Everybody told me that hath-yoga is included in bhakti-yoga and I didn't need to do *haṭha-yoga*; I only needed to dance in *kirtan.*

I was stubborn about that for a while, but when I moved in the temple, there was no time for it and no place to do it. Then when I go to be with Prabhupāda, I started doing it again. In the midmorning, before cooking for him, I went in the backyard and did some *yoga-āsanas*, but I wanted to make sure it was okay. After I'd been doing it for two or three days I had full intent to ask Prabhupāda about it that day, but when I brought his lunch plate in, he said, "I see you're dong yoga exercises in the yard." I said, "Yes sir, I was going to ask you about that. The devotees told me that that's not bona fide, it's not our process." "Actually," Prabhupāda said, "these exercises are very good for your health. We don't want anyone to become distracted, so we don't teach it. But for you, it's very good, and I encourage you to do it."

(Interview with Nanda Kumar Dāsa)

Jumping Jacks

On a light note, I was on a morning walk when one devotee asked if he should practice yoga, just for health, because he was sitting at a desk most of the day. Śrīla Prabhupāda replied "Yes. Or you can do...what is it called...?"and he made the gesture of "jumping jacks" (the exercise you often see the military or sports teams doing).

(Remembrance by Badri Nārāyaṇa Dāsa)

Prāṇāyāma

In some of the *Purāṇas* the evidence is given that if someone is simply meditating on devotional activities, he has achieved the desired result and has seen face to face the Supreme Personality of Godhead. In this connection, there is a story in the *Brahmā-vaivarta Purāṇa* that in the city of Pratiṣṭhānapura in South India there was once a *brāhmaṇa* who was not very well-to-do, but who was nevertheless satisfied in himself, thinking that it was because of his past misdeeds and by the desire of Kṛṣṇa that he did not get sufficient money and opulence. So he was not at all sorry for his poor material position, and he used to live very peacefully. He was very openhearted, and sometimes he went to hear some lectures delivered by great realized souls. At one such meeting, while he was very faithfully hearing about Vaiṣṇava activities, he was informed that these activities can be performed even by meditation. In other words, if a person is unable to actually perform Vaiṣṇava activities physically, he can meditate upon the Vaiṣṇava activities and thereby acquire all of the same results. Because the *brāhmaṇa* was not very well-to-do financially, he decided that he would simply meditate on grand, royal devotional activities, and he began this business thus:

Sometimes he would take his bath in the River Godāvari. After taking his bath he would sit in a secluded place on the bank of the river, and by practicing the yoga exercises of *prāṇāyāma*, the usual breathing exercises, he would concentrate his mind. These breathing exercises are meant to mechanically fix the mind upon a particular subject. That is the result of the breathing exercises and also of the different sitting postures of yoga. Formerly, even quite ordinary persons used to know how to fix the mind upon the remembrance of the Lord, and so the *brāhmaṇa* was doing this.

(The Nectar of Devotion, Chapter 10)

Massage and Other Things

Hints about maintaining health.

After the morning walks, Prabhupāda would take a light breakfast of fruits and then sit at his desk, sometimes closing his eyes while pleasant breezes and morning sunshine entered his room. I felt that he was using this Bombay stop to gain a little strength, after traveling and working so hard. I was glad to see him resting, since he usually rested only about four hours in twenty-four. I preferred to see Prabhupāda not giving extra lectures and meeting guests all day. The main thing, especially at his age, was to keep good health and continue his writing. So this occasional resting in the morning seemed appropriate.

For me, Prabhupāda's daily massage was the high point of the day. It was supposed to begin at eleven-fifteen in the morning, but sometimes he would be talking with guests at that time.

In that case, I would put on my *gamchā* (cloth that is used to wrap around the waist) and sit conspicuously in his audience, hoping that they would understand that it was time for his massage. Sometimes I even said, "Prabhupāda, it is time for your massage." He would sometimes ignore me, or sometimes take the hint and manage to have the audience depart. I was always concerned that he start his massage on time, otherwise his lunch would be late, and his whole afternoon schedule would be off.

He would put on his *gamchā* and sit on the veranda floor in the late morning sunshine. I would rub mustard seed oil over his body, starting with the top of his head, and he would relax, often with half-closed eyes, and allow his body to rock slightly with the movements of my massaging. It was lush in Bombay, and while sitting, Prabhupāda could see the tops of the coconut trees against the blue sky. There were nice tropical breezes, and Prabhupāda called it a paradise. "Have you ever seen such a lush place?" he asked, and he would speak of many things, but not as constantly as on the morning walk.

(Life with the Perfect Master, Chap. 5)

Climate

So far your health is concerned, Hawaii is very good climate. You can take bath in the sea, and that will keep your health. Take *dāl*, especially urad, a little cheese, peanuts, green vegetables, especially squash leaf.

(Letter to Sudāmā Dāsa, December 10, 1973)

He had some practical advice for maintaining the health of the traveling party also. "In the hot climates, hold programs at nighttime, and the daytime can be used for resting. Also, green mango sherbert can be prepared. Roast the green mango, and take out the pulp. Mix this pulp with a little salt, black pepper, sugar, and make a liquid by adding some water, then drink it. This will give protection from stroke from the heat."

(Transcendental Diary, Vol. 2, Chap. 5, June 7, 1976)

Sleeping

Sleeping on the upstairs landing just outside Śrīla Prabhupāda's quarters, I occasionally hear him come out of his room to go to the bathroom in the middle of the night. As he passes by I roll over in my sleeping bag onto my knees and offer my obeisances. Prabhupāda paused tonight and with concern asked, "So, you cannot sleep? You are suffering from insomnia?"

And then, with mild amusement, he added, "I also have the same disease." Still, it was clear he would have preferred me to sleep.

(Transcendental Diary, Vol. 2, Chap. 5, June 7, 1976)

Toothbrush

If you can find eucalyptus twigs, you can send them to me wherever I am in the world, and I shall always have nice toothbrushes thanks to you. Eucalyptus is the best.

(Letter to Dāmodara Dāsa, August 6, 1972)

Mental Health

The best cure for mental disease is to be continuously engaged in hearing and chanting about Lord Kṛṣṇa. When you understand where the root of the tree is, you can give it proper nourishment. Similarly, if you understand the root cause of a disease, you can administer the proper medicine. The real source of mental disease is a lack of awareness of the Supreme Lord.

Mental Health—Psychiatry

Psychiatrists are humbug, all humbug. They cannot help. Best thing is to be engaged in continuously chanting and hearing *sankirtana*, that will cure anyone of mental disease.

(Letter to Upendra Dāsa, February 19, 1972)

Guest (1) (young man): Would you like to give your views on psychiatry?...
Guest (1): Is it necessary to have a therapeutic system?
Prabhupāda: No, everything. First of all we have to understand that everything is expansion of God's energy. So if you understand God, then the energies are automatically understood. *Kasmin tu bhagavo vijñāte sarvam idaṁ vijñātaṁ bhavati.* This is the Vedic injunction. If you try to understand God, then His energies also will be understood by you. If you know the root, if you water on the root of the tree, then the tree, whole

tree, becomes luxuriantly flourished. So our proposition is: you take the root, Kṛṣṇa, and you will understand everything properly from the root. If you want to understand the tree, whole tree, you try to understand it from the root, not from the top. So disease, any disease, if you understand the root cause of the disease you can give proper medicine and he's cured.

So psychiatrists generally their patients are crazy fellows. Generally they treat crazy fellows. Is it not? No sane man goes to a psychiatrist. (laughter) Is it not a fact? So all these crazy men sometimes makes the psychiatrist a crazy also. So more or less, everyone is crazy. That is the... It is not my layman's opinion. It is the opinion of a big medical surgeon. There was a case in the court, murder case. The murderer pleaded that I became crazy, mad, at that time. That is generally...So the medical man was called to examine. He was great civil surgeon in Calcutta. So he gave his opinion in the court that so far I have treated many patients, so my opinion is that everyone is more or less a madman. More or less. It is a question of degree. So our opinion is like that, that anyone who is not under the direct connection with God, he's a crazy man. He's a madman. Now you can treat. So we are also psychiatrists. We are pushing this Kṛṣṇa consciousness. So because anyone who is in this material world—more or less crazy, madman. Because he doesn't care for God, therefore he's crazy. He is completely under the control of God, but still, he has the audacity to say, No, I don't believe in God. Crazy man. So anyone who does not believe in God, he's a crazy fellow. You can treat him. Everyone is patient. This crazy fellow is fully under the control of material nature, and he's still thinking that he is independent. That is craziness. Everyone is thinking like that, so everyone is a patient of psychiatrist.

"How we can declare independence? There is no independence...This is knowledge. Nobody wants to die, but nature says, 'You must die...' But the crazy fellow says, 'I am independent. I think like this.' What is the value of your thinking? You may think in your favor, but the nature will not allow you. So everyone is crazy who is declaring independence. He's a crazy."

(Lecture on Bhagavad-gitā 9.4, Melbourne, April 23, 1976)

Open Space and Fresh Air

Puṣṭa Kṛṣṇa: It's from these automobiles, the exhaust. They say that in some cities like New York, just living in the city itself, it is like smoking two packs of cigarettes every day because of so much pollution in the air, so contaminated. (break)...in the Śrīmad-Bhāgavatam that the cure for madness is open space and fresh air. That's Āyurvedic method. So in the cities there's all kinds of confined spaces, the air is not all clean. There's so much madness.

(Conversation, Los Angeles, June 8, 1976)

Every morning after breakfast Śrīla Prabhupāda goes up the back stairs and onto his roof. On the back section, overlooking his back garden, I lay out a mattress, sheet, and pillow, and he takes his morning nap lying in the sunshine. It is quiet and pleasant, the sun warming but not too strong, the air clear and the breeze gentle. Prabhupāda likes to get out in the fresh air when he can, and the roof provides a haven for him free from the constant stream of visitors and management. After about an hour he comes down again, refreshed and ready to meet the day's demands.

(Transcendental Diary, Vol. 5, Chap. 3, November 15, 1976)

Puṣṭa Kṛṣṇa picked out something interesting from [Chapter Sixteen] verse nine. He said that in the word-for-word translation the demonic are described as *prabhavanti*, they flourish, and at the same time, *kṣayāya*, which means for destruction. So this seemed to be a contradiction.

Prabhupāda explained that it means materially. "Just like when you go to a modern city and say, 'Oh, how developed,' *prabhavanti*. But what kind of *prabhavanti*? That is next word, *jagato 'hitāḥ*, to destroy this world. So their *prabhavanti* is in the opposite direction. That is not *prabhavanti* actually. *Prabhavanti* in the material sense, but what is the purpose, what is the end? There are two kinds of progress, to hell, to heaven."

I mentioned that fifty years ago people were thinking that it was progress to build big skyscrapers, but now it's so hellish in the cities that everybody is moving out.

Śrīla Prabhupāda agreed. "Yes. Actually, when there are so many skyscraper buildings, it is hell. The natural air is obstructed. In Bombay you'll see. If you are in the top floor you have got little facility, in the lower floor it is hell. If there are several skyscraper buildings, in the first floor, second floor, it is simply hell. No air. Simply you have to run on this electric fan. You cannot see the sky. Therefore it is meant skyscraper? What is scraper? What is the meaning?"

"It touches the sky," I said.

"So you have touched the sky in such a way I cannot see even. This is the result. You demon, you have captured the sky, so I have no opportunity to see even. Always electric light." He looked around the beautiful garden, through the trees and across the valleys beyond. "Now we see the sky, the sun, how nice it is. This is life. Green, down and up, clear sky, sun, this is life. We get rejuvenation in this atmosphere. What is this nonsense, all skyscraper building, no air, no light. *Jagato 'hitāḥ*. The mind becomes crippled, the health becomes deteriorated, children cannot see even the sky, everything is spoiled."

(Transcendental Diary, Vol. 3, Chap. 1, June 26, 1976)

Healthy Life with a Sound Mind

Human activities diseased by a tendency toward sense gratification have been regulated in the Vedas under the principles of salvation. This system employs religion, economic development, sense gratification and salvation, but at the present moment people have no interest in religion or salvation. They have only one aim in life — sense gratification — and in order to achieve this end they make plans for economic development.

Misguided men think that religion should be maintained because it contributes to economic development, which is required for sense gratification. Thus in order to guarantee further sense gratification after death, in heaven, there is some system of religious observance. But this is not the purpose of religion. The path of religion is actually meant for self-realization, and economic development is required just to maintain the body in a sound, healthy condition. A man should lead a healthy life with a sound mind just to realize *vidyā*, true knowledge, which is the aim of human life. This life is not meant for working like an ass or for culturing *avidyā* for sense gratification.

(Śrī Īśopaniṣad, Mantra 11, purport)

Anxiety Creates Disease

So how these people, during the time of Mahārāja Yudhiṣṭhira, were free from all kinds of anxieties and diseases? *Nädhayo vyädhayaḥ kleśāḥ*. If you are in anxiety, then that will create a disease. Our this psychological condition, physiological condition, is working in so subtle way – little shocking, little disturbance will create another disturbance. The Āyurvedic medicine, they treat patients on this principle, how things are disturbed...

So if people remain completely in hygienic principle, as they are prescribed in the *Śāstras*, just like rise early in the morning, take bath, evacuate and chant Hare Kṛṣṇa mantra... If you follow the rules and regulation, then there will be no anxiety, no disease. People become crazy when he is full of anxieties or disease. If he is happy in every respect, then he does not become crazy, he does not become enemy. If everyone is satisfied, then where is the chance of becoming your enemy or my enemy? Everyone is satisfied.

(Bhaktivedanta Lecture, Śrīmad-Bhāgavatam *1.10.6, Māyāpur, June 21 1973)*

Kulaśekhara dāsa, formerly of London, was also present. Śrīla Prabhupāda recalled how Kulaśekhara's father, a London docker, was driving for him during one of his visits. Kulaśekhara told Prabhupāda that he was finding country life to be so much more peaceful and less anxiety-ridden than living in the city.

"Yes," Prabhupāda said. "Less disease, less brain taxing. Everything is less. And if you have temple, it is very happy life. Just for your food work a little, and balance time engage yourself in Kṛṣṇa consciousness. This is ideal life."

(Transcendental Diary, Vol. 3, Chap. 1, June 24, 1976)

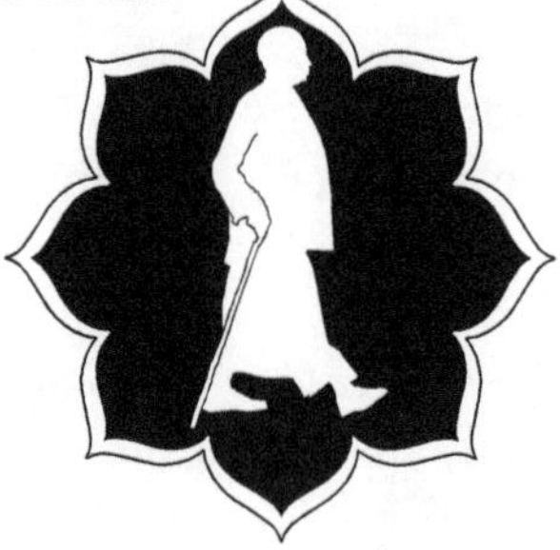

Chapter 4
Treating Disease

Treat the Root Cause

The root cause of our diseases is that we are subject to the modes of material nature. A spiritual master physician has the cure for this. Sattva-guṇa, rajo-guṇa and tamo-guṇa. These are three qualities of the material energy. Sattva is illuminating, rajo is passionate, tamo-guna, ignorance is dull and lifeless.

Just by treating the root cause of an ailment, one can conquer all bodily pains and sufferings. Similarly, if one is devoted and faithful to the spiritual master, he can conquer the influence of *sattva-guṇa*, *rajo-guṇa* and *tamo-guṇa* very easily.

(Śrīmad-Bhāgavatam 7.15.25, purport)

Bad Signs

Someone who cannot sleep immediately upon resting, and someone who passes stool immediately after eating, will very soon be called by Yamarāja. But a physician cannot make a living from someone who passes stool before a meal and urinates after.

Harikeśa is becoming increasingly ill. He looks weak and emaciated and has no strength. It is all he can do just to cook Śrīla Prabhupāda's lunch.

Prabhupāda observed him going to the toilet just after eating breakfast. He shook his head and quoted a Bengali proverb, "He who cannot sleep immediately upon resting and he who passes stool immediately after eating will very soon be called by Yamarāja . On the other hand, he who passes stool before eating and urine after, the physician cannot make a living from!"

(Transcendental Diary, Vol. 1, Chap. 9, January 25, 1976)

Birth, Death, Old Age, and Disease

Regarding the auto accident, just hold a condolence meeting for Rāghava dāsa *brahmacārī*, and pray for his soul to Kṛṣṇa for giving him a good chance for advancement in Kṛṣṇa consciousness. Certainly Kṛṣṇa will give him a good place to take birth where he can again begin in Kṛṣṇa consciousness activities. That is sure. But we offer our condolences to a departed soul separated from a Vaiṣṇava. Do you know that there must be *prasādam* distributed? After three days after the demise of a Vaiṣṇava a function should be held for offering the departed soul and all others *prasādam*. This is the system.

(Letter to Revatīnandana dāsa, November 14, 1973)

One should try to understand the distress of accepting birth, death, old age and disease. There are descriptions in various Vedic literatures of birth. In the Śrīmad-Bhāgavatam the world of the unborn, the child's stay in the womb of the mother, its suffering, etc., are all very graphically described. It should be thoroughly understood that birth is distressful. Because we forget how much distress we have suffered within the womb of the mother, we do not make any solution to the repetition of birth and death. Similarly at the time of death there are all kinds of sufferings, and they are also mentioned in the authoritative scriptures. These should be discussed. And as far as disease and old age are concerned, everyone gets practical experience. No one wants to be diseased, and no one wants to become old, but there is no avoiding these. Unless we have a pessimistic view of this material life, considering the distresses of birth, death, old age and disease, there is no impetus for our making advancement in spiritual life.

(Bhagavad-gītā 13.8-12, purport)

When the disease is there, you go to the doctor, take medicine, try to become cured from the disease. But nobody inquires that why I am subjected to this disease? That is intelligence. Precaution is better than cure. If you know how to protect yourself from disease, then that is better position than to become diseased and cured. That is not very good intelligence. Rather, don't be diseased, not that you become diseased repeatedly and go to the medical man and be cured. *Punaḥ punaś carvita-carvaṇānām*. They have been described as chewing the chewed again and again. So actually our problem is that we are diseased at the present moment, every one of us. What is that disease? *Janma-mṛtyu-jarā-vyādhi-duhkha-doṣānudarśanam*. This is our disease: we are forced to die, we are forced to take birth, we are forced to become old and we are forced to become diseased.

(Lecture on Caitanya-caritāmṛta, Madhya-līlā 20.120, Bombay, November 12, 1975)

Prabhupāda: Hm. *Kṛṣṇa tvadīya-pada-paṅkaja-pañjarāntam adyaiva me viśatu mānasa-rāja-haṁsaḥ, prāṇa-prayāṇa*...Ordinary dying, *kapha-pitta-vāyu*: *Ghara ghara ghar*, choking and...But in the *kīrtana* if we die, oh, it is so successfully... Injection, operation...Who needs it? That atmosphere death and Kṛṣṇa-*kīrtana* death? Glorious death. Oxygen gas...(laughs) Dying and so much trouble. Never be disturbed, call doctor-no. Chant Hare Kṛṣṇa. Go on chanting. You have got so much material.

(Conversation, Vrindavana, May 27, 1977)

Hari-śauri entered Śrīla Prabhupāda's room and reported the death of an Australian devotee in Bhubaneswar. He told Śrīla Prabhupāda that Saṁjāta had joined the Melbourne temple at age 51 after leaving his family life. Being an architect, he had come to India to work with Saurabha on designs for a temple in Haridaspur, and had recently been working under Gour Govinda Mahārāja in Bhubaneswar. He had contracted a virulent brain virus, his health had deteriorated rapidly and he had left his body the previous day. Hari-śauri wondered about Saṁjāta's destination after death.

"Is Bhubaneswar part of Jagannātha Purī *dhāma*?"

Prabhupāda, appearing frail and thin, was resting on the bed, but answered definitively, "Oh, yes."

"Is that a guarantee for going home, if someone leaves their body in the *dhāma*?"

"At least," Prabhupāda answered, "he gets high standard of life for many years. That is stated in the *Bhagavad-gītā*." He asked Hari-śauri to find the relevant verses in *Bhagavad-gītā*, and Hari-śauri read aloud from Chapter 6, verses 41 to 43:

"The unsuccessful yogi after many, many years of enjoyment on the planets of the pious living entities, is born into a family of righteous people or into a family of rich aristocracy, or he takes his birth in a family of transcendentalists who are surely great in wisdom. Verily, such a birth is rare in this world, and taking such a birth, he again revives the divine consciousness of his previous life, and he tries to make further progress in order to achieve complete success, O son of Kuru."

Thus Śrīla Prabhupāda confirmed Saṁjāta's auspicious future.

(Conversation, Vrindavana, October 25, 1977)

During massage time the famous magician, P. C. Sarkar came to see Prabhupāda. He showed Prabhupāda some photos and suggested that he could put on a show for the pleasure of Prabhupāda and the devotees. Prabhupāda agreed, and so at 4:00 p.m. many devotees, including the Gurukula boys, assembled in his *darśana* room.

Śrīla Prabhupāda sat behind his desk, and Mr. Sarkar stood to his left, facing his audience. Both were in a jolly mood, and for about twenty minutes Mr. Sarkar demonstrated many sleight-of-hand tricks, making coins disappear and then seemingly reappear from behind Prabhupāda's ear. We were a little unsure at him using Śrīla Prabhupāda as his stooge, but Prabhupāda laughed brightly and so we also laughed along with him.

As the show ended Śrīla Prabhupāda grinned broadly and issued his famous visitor a challenge. "Sarkarji, I am a better magician than you!"

Laughing, Mr. Sarkar asked, "Oh, how is that?"

"You can make coins disappear," Prabhupāda said, "but can you make birth, old age, disease and death disappear?"

"No Swamiji, I cannot."

"Well I can," Prabhupāda said.

With a big smile on his face, Mr. Sarkar conceded defeat. "Yes, you are definitely a better magician than me."

All the devotees cheered loudly as Śrīla Prabhupāda and his guest laughed heartily.

(Transcendental Diary, Vol. 4, Chap. 5, September 11, 1976)

A well-dressed, middle-aged Indian man stepped forward and asked, "Swamiji, what is the importance of health in life, and how do you advise people to maintain health? And how does it connect to your mission?" Prabhupāda: "What is health? First of all you have to understand that however healthy you may be, you must die. So what problem will you have solved? *Janma-mṛtyu-jarā-vyādhi duḥkha-doṣānudarśanam*, Kṛṣṇa says. It is not my manufacturing. Although you may try to remain very healthy, nature's law is that you must die. How can you help yourself? After all, you have to meet death. So long as you have got this material body, there is no question of health. You must suffer. You may be a very great scientist, but nature's law must act. *Prakṛteḥ kriyamāṇāni* (the soul is forced by material nature to perform certain activities). Foolish persons bewildered by false egotism think, 'I am improving my health, I am improving this...' He is improving nothing. He's completely under the clutches of material nature. He can't act anything independently. That is the law of nature."

(Śrīla Prabhupādā Līlāmṛta Chap. 51)

Natural Life

Purity is the force behind health.

The breathing air of life is produced of sky, air and water, and therefore open air, regular bath and ample space in which to live are favorable for healthy vitality. Fresh produce from the earth like grains and vegetables, as well as fresh water and heat, is good for the upkeep of the gross body.

(Śrīmad-Bhāgavatam 2.10.31, purport)

Holy Place

A special place for health.

In the *Caitanya-Bhāgavāta* (*Antya-khaṇḍa*, Chapter Two) it is said that when Lord Śrī Caitanya Mahāprabhu arrived at Śrī Bhuvaneśvara, He visited the temple of Lord Śiva known as Gupta-Kāśī (the concealed Väräṇasī). Lord Siva established this as a place of pilgrimage by bringing water from all holy places and creating the lake known as Bindu-sarovara. Śrī Caitanya Mahāprabhu took His bath in this lake, feeling a great regard for Lord Śiva. From the spiritual point of view, people still go to take a bath in this lake. Actually, by taking a bath there, one becomes very healthy even from the material viewpoint. Taking a bath and drinking the water of this lake can cure any disease of the stomach. Regular bathing certainly cures indigestion.

(Caitanya-caritāmṛta, Madhya-lilā 5.141, purport)

Consult Approved Physician

To cure disease, follow an approved method and rely upon Lord Kṛṣṇa.

Regarding Śyāmā dāsī's health, it is to be understood that so long as we have got this material body there must be some trouble. Actually, medicine is not the remedial measures for our bodily troubles unless we are helped by Kṛṣṇa. Therefore, whenever there is bodily trouble we may adopt the prescribed methods of medical science and depend upon Kṛṣṇa for His Mercy. The best remedy, not only for Śyāmā dāsī but for everyone, is to consult some approved physician. But ultimately we have to depend on the Mercy of Kṛṣṇa, so we should chant regularly, pray to Kṛṣṇa to give us a chance to serve Him, and, if required, we may adopt the approved method of treatment.

(Letter to Kīrtanānanda Swami, February 14, 1969)

Control the Discharge of Semen

Controlling the discharge of semen means conquering the problem of death.

After this, semen (the faculty of procreation) and the god who presides over the waters appeared. Next appeared an anus and then the organs of defecation and thereupon the god of death, who is feared throughout the universe.

(Śrīmad-Bhāgavatam 3.26.57)

It is understood herewith that the faculty to discharge semen is the cause of death. Therefore, yogis and transcendentalists who want to live for greater spans of life voluntarily restrain themselves from discharging semen. The more one can restrain the discharge of semen, the more one can be aloof from the problem of death. There are many yogis living up to three hundred or seven hundred years by this process, and in the *Bhāgavatam* it is clearly stated that discharging semen is the cause of horrible death. The more one is addicted to sexual enjoyment, the more susceptible he is to a quick death.

(Śrīmad-Bhāgavatam 3.26.57, purport)

Deafness

Deafness is not an impediment for advancing in Kṛṣṇa consciousness.

With regard to your son, let him see the Deity and ask him to offer obeisances. He will see and learn it. Yes, the body is received according to karma, still it is not an impediment to advance in Kṛṣṇa consciousness by being deaf. Just teach him to see the Deity and how to offer obeisances and he will take *prasādam*. These things will elevate him to Kṛṣṇa consciousness. Later on if Kṛṣṇa desires, he can develop his hearing power. Kṛṣṇa is almighty and He can do whatever He likes. What is the use of the *karmī* deaf school. Better to sit him down before the Deity and see and offer obeisances.

(Letter to Locanānanda Dāsa and Rameśvarī Dāsī, November 9, 1975)

Doctors

A devotee who is a preacher is a first-class doctor, and he or she can help you cure the soul's disease in this material world. One who is trained by a bona fide doctor can also become a bona fide doctor. If you have a disease, go to a doctor, but don't ask blessings from a saintly person to cure your illness.

Regarding your proposal to become a doctor, because your mother wants to prosecute your education, I think if you can learn Kṛṣṇa consciousness perfectly, by reading our different literatures, and books, you will be a better doctor than the ordinary physician. The ordinary physician may cure the disease of the body, but if you become advanced in Kṛṣṇa consciousness, you will be able to cure the disease of the soul for many many persons. And that is more important than a doctor or medical practitioner for curing the disease of this body. However we may be expert for keeping this body fit, it is sure and certain that this will end. But if you can protect the soul from being fallen a victim of this material existence that is a greater service. In some of the Vedic literatures, it is said that *atmanan sarvato rakṣet*, that means one should give first protection to the soul. Then he should take care of his particular type of faith, then he should take care of the material things, namely this body, and anything in relation with this body, or wealth. Please try to read all our books very carefully, and whenever there is any doubt, you ask me, and be expert preacher. That will make you a great doctor for protecting the human society from being fallen a victim to *māyā*. I hope this will meet you in good health.

(Letter to Toṣaṇa Kṛṣṇa Dāsa, Seattle, October 7, 1968)

Tamāl Kṛṣṇa: His idea is that if one receives a mantra from a spiritual master, if the spiritual master is not bona fide…

Prabhupāda: Then there is no question of mantra. There is no question of worshiping Deity. These are all bogus things. If you are not… Just like here is a young medical man. If he has not received instruction from a bona fide medical college, so what is the value of his medical, being… That is… What is called? What is the technical name?

Devotee(4): Quack.

Prabhupāda: Quack! (laughter)(pronounces like quack)

Devotees: Quack.

Prabhupāda: A quack is not a medical man, however he may show all red bottles, white bottles. There is a Bengali proverb, *naj jal yac curi tini ei daktar*. One stethoscope, *naj*, and some bottles, *jala*, and talking all nonsense, he becomes a doctor. That means the quack doctor, not a… Qualified doctor, he knows what is what. So *naj jal yac curi tini ei daktar*. In Bengali they say. And mostly in villages they go on like that. But of course, they have got some experience. I know in Allahabad there was a doctor, Kabhir, a Dr. Kabhir. And because in my previous household life I was a chemist and druggist, I was supplying medicine, so he was my customer. So he had very, very big prac... He was my biggest customer. He was purchasing medicine like anything. But he had experience. He learned from an experienced doctor. He cannot be called a bogus, because whatever he learned, he was... But generally, one who is not a bona fide doctor, he is called a quack. So anything, experience required, not that you have to go to the medical college. If you are trained under a bona fide doctor, then also you can get the quality of a doctor.

(Lecture on Śrīmad-Bhāgavatam 6.1.41–42,
Surat, December 23, 1970)

To contrast this genuine mood of associating with a saintly person, Śrīla Prabhupāda made an amusing indirect reference to an incident on the train to Nellore on January 3rd of this year, when he was approached by some gentlemen for benedictions.

"Not that simply asking, 'Give me your blessing.' And 'Why? Are you worthy for blessing?' Cheap blessing. And blessing also – they do not know what is blessing. Blessing, they think that 'I have got some disease; if the saintly person gives me some blessing, I will be relieved from this disease.' Now why don't you go to the doctor? But you go to saintly person for curing your disease. This is *anyābhilāṣitā*, that they do not know even how to approach a saintly person.

(Transcendental Diary, Vol. 5, Chap. 3, October 31, 1976)

Dispensary

So, if people become interested in our philosophy, then we shall consider the other two items, namely, the nursery school and dispensary. So far dispensary is concerned, we have none all over the world. It will be a new attempt. So far the school is concerned, we have got in Africa and America, and we have got men experienced to teach on our line. But for dispensary, we have no experience at all."

(Letter to Dr. Ghosh, April 5, 1975)

The Holy Names

The proper medicine is chanting Hare Kṛṣṇa, and the proper food is Kṛṣṇa prasāda.

If you are feeling tired, you may take rest. Your body is very valuable. It is dedicated to Kṛṣṇa, so you must take care of the body very carefully. The best medicine is to rest and chant the Hare Kṛṣṇa mantra, along with the doctor's prescription. The Hare Kṛṣṇa mantra is *bhavauṣadhi*, the panacea for all material disease.

(Letter to Girirāja dāsa, August 12, 1971)

So far your other letter, devotion does not depend on the body, and in spite of all difficulties we can chant, so long we have got the tongue—and even we have got no tongue we can chant in our mind. So where is the question of not serving with devotion? On the contrary, I consider that you and your good husband, Gaurasundara, are two of my topmost disciples and the work you are doing greatly encourages and pleases me, therefore do not think that because you are sometimes sick or weak that you are not making any advancement and that you are disappointing me, no. I am always thinking upon you both, that Kṛṣṇa will give you His all blessings. Simply if you are able always to chant Hare Kṛṣṇa, that is the same as following all other regulative principles.

(Letter to Govinda Dāsī, February 12, 1972)

So in our, this human form of life we should be very careful, and what is ordered that You should do like this... Just like if you go to a medical man, so if you are diseased, a medical man, physician, will give you a prescription that You take this medicine, and you do not take this kind of food. You can take this kind of food. *Āhāra-pathya*. So if you want to cure your material disease, then two things are required: the medicine and the food. It is called *pathya*. The proper food and proper medicine. The proper medicine is chanting Hare Kṛṣṇa, and the proper food is Kṛṣṇa *prasāda*.

*(Lecture on Śrīmad-*Bhāgavatam *6.1.42, Los Angeles, June 8, 1976)*

Pālikā dāsī was once very ill, and although doctors had prescribed mudpacks from the Yamuna and other remedies, she remained in a critical condition. A devotee described to Prabhupāda Pālikā dāsī's symptoms.

Prabhupāda said she should take *caraṇāmṛta* and that two women devotees should alternate chanting Hare Kṛṣṇa right next to Pālikā all day and night. Pālikā dāsī was cured by this treatment.

(Śrīla Prabhupāda Nectar, Vol. 5, No. 13)

There was no morning walk today. Missing Prabhupāda on the beach, Dr. Patel arrived at his apartment with his son. He took a cardiograph reading and gave Prabhupāda some pills. His diagnosis is high blood pressure. Prabhupāda rested. He didn't take breakfast, and then ate only a morsel at lunch, complaining of dizziness from the medicine. He remarked that modern drugs are medicines for the demons. Prabhupāda rarely goes to a doctor, although if by some arrangement one comes to him, he doesn't refuse their help. Disease has to be treated, of course, but as far as he is concerned, chanting Hare Kṛṣṇa is the best cure.

(Transcendental Diary, Vol. 1, Chap. 4, December 21, 1975)

Take Rest If Sick

If you're sick, it's sometimes necessary to take complete rest.

I have received your letter dated January 28, 1969 regarding Jadurāṇī's sick health. She requires complete rest. All of her work should be suspended and she should be given liquid foods, just like barley water mixed with milk. Purchase pearl barley from the market, and the recipe is 1 cup of barley and 4 cups of water to be boiled for at least one half hour. That liquid preparation may be mixed with milk and sugar and she may take. Jadurāṇī must not exert herself in any way. She should take complete rest and chant Hare Kṛṣṇa. When she next wants to begin work, she must take my permission. For the time being, all work must be suspended.

(Letter to Satsvarūpa Dāsa, January 31, 1969)

The most concerning part of your letter is about your health. You write to say that by 3 o'clock in the evening you get a slight fever, and your head begins to ache, and you feel tired and wish to take rest. This is not a very good sign. The immediate program is that you will have to be relieved from these symptoms. So the first thing is that you should take complete rest. So far as New York is concerned, I don't think different engagement there will allow you to take rest. I would have advised you to go to New Vṛndāvana immediately but it is cold there like New York. Under the circumstances, if you like to come here and take rest you are welcome. But wherever you like you may take rest and not be strained at all. That is my opinion, and I shall be glad to know what you are going to do in this connection.

(Letter to Rāyarāma Dāsa, February 20, 1969)

So far as getting engagements, don't expect any help from Sadānanda because I understand he is practically ruined by his health. So don't trouble him, and let him take full rest.

(Letter to Kṛṣṇa Dāsa, May 17, 1969)

I am sorry to learn that your health is not very good at the present time. The best thing is that you rest for some time until you are feeling stronger. When Jadurāṇī was feeling very weak, I advised her to take complete rest until she was stronger and then I advised her to go out on *saṅkīrtana* party. So you may follow the same procedure of taking as much rest as you feel you require, and then when you feel it is all right, you resume your activities.

(Letter to Madana Dāsa, Los Angeles, July 23, 1969)

If Kṛṣṇa devī is continuing to feel weakness she may reduce any strenuous activity and increase the number of rounds chanting. I hope her heath has improved by now.

(Letter to Dinesh Dāsa, January 22, 1970)

If you are feeling tired, you may take rest. Your body if very valuable. It is dedicated to Kṛṣṇa, so you must take care of the body very carefully. The best medicine is to rest and chant the Hare Kṛṣṇa mantra, along with the doctor's prescription. The Hare Kṛṣṇa mantra is: *bhavauṣadhi*, the panacea for all material disease.

(Letter to Girirāja Dāsa, August 12, 1971)

Regarding the Nārāyaṇa Kavaca mantra (certain recitations for protection), the Hare Kṛṣṇa mantra is everything. But, I think that you are working to hard. Your illness is the result of too hard work. Remain in Māyāpur. Take rest as much as necessary. And work through your assistants. And chant Hare Kṛṣṇa.

(Letter to Jayapatāka Swami, December 4, 1976)

Proper and Practical

Do whatever is required and most practical to treat a disease.

Regarding your physical malady, you should do whatever is required to treat it properly. Whatever is most practical.

(Letter to Bhakta Dāsa, May 7, 1975)

Illness and Remedies

Śrīla Prabhupāda gives some suggested remedies for illnesses.

Ailment of the Finger

Regarding the ailments with your finger, I am describing here a treatment for it. Take turmeric powder and add the same quantity of limestone. Then mix with water and boil it to a paste. Then apply the paste while it is hot. I understand that Hayagrīva had some backache so for him you take one part of a crushed to a powder red pepper and add to it five parts of rubbing alcohol. Keep this for 24 hours, then strain and add one part camphor. When it is mixed, just apply it on the painful part of the back 3 times daily.

(Letter to Shyāma Dāsī, February 21, 1969)

Antiseptic

Cow dung is antiseptic.

But this bone of an animal, conch shell, is pure. Just like sometimes our students are perplexed when we say that onion is not to be taken, but onion is a vegetable. So *Śabda-pramāṇa* means the Vedic evidence should be taken in such a way that no argument. There is meaning; there is no contradiction. There is meaning. Just like several times I have told you that cow dung. Cow dung is, according to Vedic injunction, is pure. In India it is actually used as antiseptic. In villages especially, there is large quantity of cow dung, and they're all over the house they have smeared to make the house antiseptic. And actually after smearing cow dung in your room, when it is dried, you'll find refreshed, everything antiseptic. It is practical experience. And one Dr. Ghosa, a great chemist, he examined cow dung, that why cow dung is so much important in the Vedic literature? He found that cow dung contains all the antiseptic properties. In Āyurveda, cow dung dried and burned into ashes is used as toothpowder.

(Lecture on Bhagavad-gītā, Los Angeles, November 27, 1968)

Child Kṛṣṇa was thoroughly washed with cow urine and then smeared with the dust raised by the movements of the cows. Then different names of the Lord were applied with cow dung on twelve different parts of His body, beginning with the forehead, as done in applying *tilaka*. In this way, the child was given protection.

(Śrīmad-Bhāgavatam 10.6.20)

Appetite

In 1976 in Toronto Pāllikā was cooking for Śrīla Prabhupāda who had a toothache and had lost his appetite. Śrīla Prabhupāda instructed Pāllikā one evening to cook kacoris (a fried savory made with urad *dāl* (*dāl* high in protein) or vegetable filling) in the same way Bali Madan had made for him one day in the late 1960's. This meant to mashed urad *dāl* balls rolled in salt, hing (pungent spice), chili powder, and powdered *saunf* (anise seed/fennel). This mixture is then fried in ghee. The ghee was to stimulate taste. All the ingredients used were to help his digestion.

(B. B. Govinda Mahārāja)

Asthma

For asthma, no food should be taken at night, and in general avoid overloading the stomach. Chanting Hare Kṛṣṇa and drinking only *caraṇāmṛta* water is the best remedy for any bodily disease. But if something else required, chew a little thyme after meals. Potassium iodine is a temporary medicine for asthma.

(Letter to Upendra Dāsa, December 8, 1971)

Bleeding

I remember from Toronto that if we cut ourselves when using a knife, it was said that Prabhupāda suggested to lightly cover the cut with red chili powder to stop the bleeding.

(B. B. Govinda Mahārāja)

Cancer

You accept these principles of life, no meat-eating, no intoxication, no illicit sex, and there will be no cancer. Those who are strictly on this line, they never suffer from cancer or any such disease. Now take for example me. I've come here in this country for the last eight years. How many times have I gone to the doctor? That one heart attack. That is serious, that is another thing. Otherwise, generally how many times have I gone? I don't pay any bill of doctor. So if we live a very hygienic life, regulated life, there is no question of cancer or any disease. The disease is created by violating nature's law. One of the causes of cancer disease is this contraceptive method. You can make research on it. So they are on one side discovering contraceptive method, contraceptive chemicals, and on the other side researching for cancer disease. And they say also smoking is one of the causes. So why not give up smoking and illicit sex, contraceptive method?

(Morning Walk, Los Angeles, May 4, 1973)

Childbirth

Lāḍḍu (a sweet) made from fenugreek for recovering strength after childbirth.

(B. B. Govinda Mahārāja)

Colds

One can warm mustard oil in a *katori* (small frying pan) and rub the oil on the feet one catches cold. In 1975 when Śrīla Prabhupāda visited Toronto he had a slight cold and chill. He requested that white poppy seed, *posta dana*, be soaked and pasted, then stirred in the vegetable *chaunch* (a cooking method in which spices are added to vegetables). He said this would cause retention of heat in the body. He also requested corn on the cob, covered with aluminum foil and baked in the oven. Again for heat retention. Hot *jalebi* (fried sweet) and hot *halavā* for the cure of cold.

(B. B. Govinda Mahārāja)

Conception

Tejyas asked Śrīla Prabhupāda what to do about his problem having an erection in order to conceive of his first child. Śrīla Prabhupāda suggested eating garlic for some days prior to the *garbhādāna* (purification ceremony that householders perform before conceiving a child). It worked.

(B. B. Govinda Swami)

Diarrhea

Fresh roasted and crushed cumin seed mixed in yogurt.

(B. B. Govinda Swami)

Dry Skin

You may try using oil on the dry skin before taking your bath each day, and this may help the situation. Mustard oil, olive oil, or some sort of oil will suffice.

(Letter to Prabhāvati Dāsī, March 24, 1969)

Dysentery

In 1974 or 1975, Śrīla Prabhupāda was in Vrindavan for Janmāṣṭamī. He had blood dysentery. He requested, "Purī hot out of the ghee." This stopped his dysentery. I mentioned this to an Āyurvedic doctor, Tanmay Gosvāmī, and he said this would have lowered *vāta* and expedited recovery.

(B. B. Govinda Mahārāja)

Headache

Regarding your headaches, your bowels are not clear. This is the cause of the problem. So you should take more milk and fruits, and eat less wheat and rice. If sandalwood oil is available, you try to massage it on your shaved head. Let me know how this trouble is improving. A *brahmacārī* should not have any complaint of bodily disease.

(Letter to Toṣaṇa Kṛṣṇa Dāsa, February 17, 1969)

Put a little black pepper in a teaspoon cover it with water and slightly boiled it. Then pat it on the forehead.

(B. B. Govinda Mahārāja)

Heat Stroke

In the hot climates, hold programs at night-time, and the day-time can be used for resting. Also, green mango sherbet can be prepared. Roast the green mango, and take out the pulp. Mix this pulp with a little salt, black pepper, sugar, and make a liquid by adding some water, then drink it. This will give protection from stroke from the heat.

(Letter to Gargamuni Dāsa, June 7, 1976)

High Fever

According to Āyurvedic treatment, it is said that if one has a high fever, someone should splash him with water after gargling this water. In this way the fever subsides. Although Bharata Mahārāja was very aggrieved due to the separation of his so-called son, the deer, he thought that the moon was splashing gargled water on him from its mouth and that this water would subdue his high fever, which was raging due to separation from the deer.

(Śrīmad-Bhāgavatam 5.8.25, purport)

Infection

You have got some infection, and I am very much anxious about your cyst pain. I do not know what is the actual position but if it is ordinary, then I think a little painting of Sloan's Liniment may reduce the painful reaction. But if it is within the skin then you have to consult some physician, but you can try applying Sloan's Liniment and before applying the liniment you can foment it by heating some soft pad in hot water and apply on the spot. After heating you can apply Sloan's Liniment. I hope you will be feeling better soon. Please keep me informed.

(Letter to Gargamuni Dāsa, May 5, 1968)

Intestines and Arteries

When there was a desire to have food and drink, the abdomen and the intestines and also the arteries became manifested. The rivers and seas are the source of their sustenance and metabolism.

(Śrīmad-Bhāgavatam 2.10.29)

The controlling deities of the intestines are the rivers, and those of the arteries, the seas. Fulfillment of the belly with food and drink is the cause of sustenance, and the metabolism of the food and drink replaces the waste of the bodily energies. Therefore, the body's health is dependent on healthy actions of the intestines and the arteries. The rivers and the seas, being the controlling deities of the two, keep the intestines and the arteries in healthy order.

(Śrīmad-Bhāgavatam 2.10.29, purport)

Irregularity in Hunger and Thirst

Next grew feelings of hunger and thirst, and in their wake came the manifestation of the oceans. Then a heart became manifest, and in the wake of the heart the mind appeared.

(Śrīmad-Bhāgavatam 3.26.60)

The ocean is considered to be the presiding deity of the abdomen, where the feelings of hunger and thirst originate. When there is an irregularity in hunger and thirst, one is advised, according to Āyurvedic treatment, to take a bath in the ocean.

(Śrīmad-Bhāgavatam 3.26.60, purport)

Jaundice and Liver Disease

On arrival in Delhi I received a letter and I request you to take proper care of Gargamuni. Let him take complete rest and give him rock candy as advised above. For a diseased person suffering for jaundice, rock candy will be just appreciated and as soon as he regains health the original taste will be appreciated. As soon as it is so the patient is understood to be cured.

(Letter to Brahmānanda Dāsa, September 15, 1967)

I was very much anxious about your illness, but I've received news from Brahmānanda that you are improving. Now whatever condition it may be I advise you to take rock candy as much as possible, always keep a piece in your mouth. So far as eating is concerned you can take ripe papaya as much as you can, also if possible boil green papaya, this will be your diet and medicine. Besides this take sufficient rest and chant Hare Kṛṣṇa. So long as we have got this material body we have to undergo these situations. If we increase our love for Kṛṣṇa we shall be able to get out of this *māyā*...

You will be cured very soon rest assured, but after you get out of this diseased condition please keep fit with regular habits at least once a day take your bath and timely, eat, drink and sleep. Now you are a married man you have facility for sex life, but also this should be regulated. Increased Kṛṣṇa consciousness will reduce the propensity of sense gratification and too much sense gratification is the cause of obtaining material bodies. So there may not be bodily disturbance still it is necessary to maintain a regulated life and easily prosecute our Kṛṣṇa consciousness. I shall pray to Kṛṣṇa for your quick recovery.

(Letter to Gargamuni Dāsa, September 15, 1967)

If you take green bananas, peel them and put them out in the sun to dry for one, two, three days—till it is dry—then these may be sent to me, especially when I go to Europe. This is a very good tonic for liver, and I am now having these unripened bananas daily in Los Angeles.

(Letter to Govinda Dāsī, August 17, 1969)

The bull and the cow are the symbols of the most offenseless living beings because even the stool and urine of these animals are utilized to benefit human society.

(Śrīmad-Bhāgavatam 1.17.13, purport)

The urine of a cow is salty, and according to Āyurvedic medicine the cow's urine is very effective in treating patients suffering from liver trouble.

(Śrīmad-Bhāgavatam 3.2.8, purport)

Over the phone Radhaballabha reported that Rāmeśvara Mahārāja is very sick with hepatitis. He has seen an Āyurvedic physician who prescribed a diet of rice and mung bean juice.

When Prabhupāda heard this he said, "Who is that rascal so-called Āyurvedic doctor?" Instead he prescribed rock candy (dissolved in water if he cannot suck it) and different preparations made from green papayas. Puṣṭa Kṛṣṇa Mahārāja included this advice in his letter.

(Transcendental Diary, Vol. 2, Chap. 4, May 6, 1976)

"The devotees here in Bombay want to know what is the best way to serve *prasādam* in the temple."

"The best way," said Prabhupāda, "is in batches of twelve. Twelve sit down, and they are served hot fresh rice, *dāl*, *capātīs*, and when they are finished they wash, and another twelve sit down. That way everything is hot and fresh. It is nutritious and palatable. Eat substantially and keep your health, but not voraciously."

Then I came down with hepatitis. Paṇḍitjī had come down with it a week before me, and he would regularly talk about it with Śrīla Prabhupāda, telling him about his symptoms, his special diet, and medicine. One day Paṇḍitjī approached His Divine Grace and told him he was now passing white stool.

Śrīla Prabhupāda replied, "I also sometimes have symptoms, but I don't say anything about it. Sometimes I see the stool is white, and I think, 'This is going on.' Then it will again be reddish. Just like now I am feeling some swollen condition in my foot. But I don't talk about it. The Vaiṣṇava avoids too much emphasis on his body." With this as a warning, I tried not to dwell on my disease or allow it to cause inconvenience to Prabhupāda. But when Prabhupāda heard about it, he recommended I take sugar cane juice and also *karela* (bitter vegetable). He said maybe my illness was due to overwork. I couldn't figure out why Prabhupāda said that I was overworking, since my workload in Bombay had become light. Of course, my mind was overworking with its pro-and-con deliberations, but I wasn't sure whether he was referring to that.

(Life With the Perfect Master, Satsvarūpa Dāsa Gosvāmī: Chapter Five)

Bhakti Caru Swami tells the story of being instructed in cooking by Śrīla Prabhupāda in Rishikesh/Haridwar in 1977. He personally showed Bhakti Caru Swami how to prepare a vegetable which was practically covered in mustard oil and had 5 or 6 fully dried red chilis to be included in the small pot.

Bhakti Caru Swami cooked the preparation and Śrīla Prabhupāda ate it with relish.

The next day, he requested the same vegetable. Bhakti Caru Swami did everything the same, but reduced the amount of chili as he felt it would be detrimental to Prabhupāda's health. He served the *prasāda*, but after Śrīla Prabhupāda tasted the preparation he chastised Bhakti Caru Swami.

He told Bhakti Caru Swami that when using so much oil, a large amount of chili is necessary to stimulate the liver for digestion. Otherwise, eating oil or ghee without chili is detrimental to the health.

(B. B. Govinda Mahārāja)

Nervous Instability

The action of the air is exhibited in movements, mixing, allowing approach to the objects of sound and other sense perceptions, and providing for the proper functioning of all other senses.

(Śrīmad-Bhāgavatam 3.26.37)

We can perceive the action of the air when the branches of a tree move or when dry leaves on the ground collect together. Similarly, it is only by the action of the air that a body moves, and when the air circulation is impeded, many diseases result.

Paralysis, nervous breakdowns, madness and many other diseases are actually due to an insufficient circulation of air. In the Āyurvedic system these diseases are treated on the basis of air circulation. If from the beginning one takes care of the process of air circulation, such diseases cannot take place. From the *Āyurveda* as well as from the Śrīmad-Bhāgavatam it is clear that so many activities are going on internally and externally because of air alone, and as soon as there is some deficiency in the air circulation, these activities cannot take place. Here it is clearly stated, *netṛtvaṁ dravya-śabdayoḥ*. Our sense of proprietorship over action is also due to the activity of the air. If the air circulation is stifled, we cannot approach a place after hearing. If someone calls us, we hear the sound because of the air circulation, and we approach that sound or the place from which the sound comes. It is clearly said in this verse that these are all movements of the air. The ability to detect odors is also due to the action of the air.

(Śrīmad-Bhāgavatam 3.26.37, purport)

The veins of the universal body became manifested and thereafter the red corpuscles, or blood. In their wake came the rivers (the deities presiding over the veins), and then appeared an abdomen.

(Śrīmad-Bhāgavatam 3.26.59)

Blood veins are compared to rivers; when the veins were manifested in the universal form, the rivers in the various planets were also manifested. The controlling deity of the rivers is also the controlling deity of the nervous system. In Āyurvedic treatment, those who are suffering from the disease of nervous instability are recommended to take a bath by dipping into a flowing river.

(Śrīmad-Bhāgavatam 3.26.59, purport)

Rheumatism

I have sent some drawings to Yamunā Devī for the certificates, and I hope she is taking proper care. I understand Mālatī is having some rheumatic condition, and it is causing pain and numbness. The best thing is to take hot baths, and massage with camphor oil, and if it is too much painful, use Sloan's Liniment. Best thing is to consult with some expert physician. The Āyurvedic medicine which I could recommend is probably not available in London, but if there is any Āyurvedic shop let me know and I shall recommend some medicine. The best thing is to chant Hare Kṛṣṇa loudly.

(Letter to Śyāmasundara Dāsa, Seattle, October 10, 1968)

Sore Throat

It was early 1968 in Los Angeles. Śyāmasundara prabhu was carving the third of four sets of *Jagannātha* deities that he would carve (the first being San Francisco, the second being New York City, fourth being London). I was also present, pregnant and not feeling well with a fever-sore throat that had lingered for three days. It was decided I should see a doctor and an appointment was secured for the afternoon. I sat by the open back door of the temple while Śyāmasundara was carving in the pleasant morning sun. *Śrīla Prabhupāda* came by to check on Shyāmasundara's progress and he inquired of my health. I explained I had fever and sore throat and would see a doctor later in the day. He replied by giving me a simple formula of hot water and salt to gargle, telling me that there was no need to see a doctor. I followed his prescription and was 'cured' by the following morning. I've followed this ever since with success.

(Mālatī devī dāsī)

Syphilis and Venereal Disease

The *kṛpaṇā bahu-duḥkha-bhājaḥ* [pain suffered by people who cannot control their senses], they know after the sex I'll have to meet so many botherations, either illicit or licit sex. Either you get so many diseases, syphilis and this, and from syphilis so many other disease, up to madness, up to leprosy, one disease after one disease, one disease. This sex...The sex syphilitic disease is called in India by the Āyurvedic physician as *phairāṅga -roga*. It has come from the Western country. I do not wish to discuss, but the point is that illicit sex has many, many aftereffects who is not very nice.

*(Lecture on Śrīmad-*Bhāgavatam *7.9.39, Māyāpur, March 17, 1976)*

Still it is in Europe and America. And now it is spreading all over. And in Āyurveda it is said, *phairāṅga*. The Europeans are described in Vedic literatures as *phairingi*, their name is *phairingi*. So this syphilitic disease is mentioned in the Āyurveda, the disease brought by the *phairingis*. And the doctor says that originally it was spread through dog. The unmarried girls, they keep dog for sex. You do not know? He knows. You will find very beautiful girl is keeping very big dog. They are trained to have sex life. And that is cause of syphilis. The dog is full of syphilitic germs. It is called *phairāṅga* in the Āyurveda. And one who has got syphilitic germs, his life is doomed. Unless it is properly treated and cured. So many disease will follow. So many. This craziness is also due to syphilitic poison, parents.

(*Lecture on Śrīmad*-Bhāgavatam 2.9.9, *Tokyo, April 25, 1972)*

Viṣṇujana: So they classify us like that. They say, You Hare Kṛṣṇa people, you want to take us back to cholera and dysentery and everything.
Prabhupāda: But you are already suffering from cancer. What you have done? (laughter) Instead of cholera, you have got cancer. Is that very good exchange?
Viṣṇujana: One out of eight men has venereal disease.
Prabhupāda: From frying pan to the fire. Cholera has got some remedy, but here there is no remedy. Hm? What is that?
Viṣṇujana: In this country they have the venereal disease. One out of ten men is suffering gonorrhea.
Prabhupāda: Yes. Long ago one professor, medical professor, he said, he was Englishman – that in our country, 75% students are suffering from venereal disease. Colonel Megor (?). Yes. Colonel Megor. There must be venereal disease because sex life is so cheap. There must be venereal disease. And venereal disease, once infected, it brings so many other diseases, one after another, one after another. The cancer is also due to that. Madness. Yes. And the Vedic civilization knew it. Therefore first restriction: Sex. *Brahmacārī*. First beginning, *brahmacārī*. No sex life. You see? Just to save. This venereal disease is mentioned in the *Āyurveda*. It is called *phiraṅgāmaya*. *Phiraṅga* means white Europeans. It is diseased... And medical science also says that it was begun from dog. The girls, they have sex life with dog and there is the beginning of venereal disease.

(Morning Walk, Los Angeles, December 31, 1973)

Toothache

For your toothache trouble, you can brush your teeth with the following mixture: common salt, one part, and pure mustard oil, quite sufficient to make it a suitable paste. With this paste brush your teeth, especially the painful part, very nicely. Gargle in hot water, and keep always some cloves in your mouth. I think this will cure your troubles. It doesn't require to extract any teeth.

(Letter to Kīrtanānanda, February 14, 1969)

Whooping Cough

Prabhupāda: Supply large quantity of milk? No.
Guest: No, that milk is medicinally used for whooping cough. Anybody suffering from whooping cough, they have to take this camel's milk. And any children who do not increase their height, they are given this milk in winter. So height is automatically increased. They become like camel eventually. (laughter) Tall, I mean. I don't mean the..., in Western way. According to Āyurvedic principle, every animal have got a particular method of curing particular disease.
Prabhupāda: Yes.

(Morning Walk Vrindavana, April 23, 1975)

Worms

In Vrindavan in 1977, many devotees had worms. When asked what to do, Prabhupāda suggested keeping a white onion when taking *prasāda* and slicing the fresh onion on the *subji*. We all ate together at that time, and I can remember how curious it was to see devotee slicing onions on what I had cooked. It worked.

(B. B. Govinda Swami)

Quick Treatment

Tamāla Kṛṣṇa: Okay, Another thing I see on account of the fast. One of the reasons perhaps...One of the advantages of fasting is that the swelling is...Fasting cures diseases.
Prabhupāda: Diet treatment is very good.

Tamāla Kṛṣṇa: That's a difficult treatment for the Westerners. Because they have no self-...
Prabhupāda: They want to be cured immediately. Go to the doctor. "Give me injection, give me tablet, cure me immediately." That is the Western treatment. Immediately stop it. Here also. A man, a worker, he's earning twenty rupees a day, and the doctors also take advantage of this rational. "You want to be treated quickly or let...?" And naturally he will say "Quickly." Then you have to take injection. Injection means each injection at least five rupees. He may inject water.

(Conversation, Bombay, April 10, 1977)

Kinds of Treatments

Śrīla Prabhupāda comments on different kinds of treatment. Generally, he preferred massage and Āyurveda.

Āyurveda

General

I may inform you that I am inclined towards Āyurvedic treatment. You can consult with the Āyurvedic physician in Vrindavan who is a Gauḍīya Vaiṣṇava...Two things are to be done if it is possible: to send me proper medicines and directions, that will be nice. But if I require to return that also I can do. Consult necessary physicians and let me know what I am to do...In Mathurā there are undoubtedly many Āyurvedic physicians and many quacks also. Try to avoid the quacks.

(Letter to Hari Bhakti Nudāsa, June 1, 1967)

The Lord in His incarnation of Dhanvantari very quickly cures the diseases of the ever-diseased living entities simply by His fame personified, and only because of Him do the demigods achieve long lives. Thus the Personality of Godhead becomes ever glorified. He also exacted a share from the sacrifices, and it is He only who inaugurated the medical science or the knowledge of medicine in the universe.

(Śrīmad-Bhāgavatam 2.7.21)

As stated in the beginning of the *Śrīmad*-Bhāgavatam, everything emanates from the ultimate source of the Personality of Godhead; it is therefore understood in this verse that medical science or knowledge in medicine was also inaugurated by the Personality of Godhead in His incarnation Dhanvantari, and thus the knowledge is recorded in the Vedas.

The Vedas are the source of all knowledge, and thus knowledge in medical science is also there for the perfect cure of the diseases of the living entity. The embodied living entity is diseased by the very construction of his body. The body is the symbol of diseases. The disease may differ from one variety to another, but disease must be there just as there is birth and death for everyone. So, by the grace of the Personality of Godhead, not only are diseases of the body and mind cured, but also the soul is relieved of the constant repetition of birth and death. The name of the Lord is also called *bhavauṣadhi*, or the source of curing the disease of material existence.

(Śrīmad-Bhāgavatam *2.7.21, purport)*

We can perceive the action of the air when the branches of a tree move or when dry leaves on the ground collect together. Similarly, it is only by the action of the air that a body moves, and when the air circulation is impeded, many diseases result. Paralysis, nervous breakdowns, madness and many other diseases are actually due to an insufficient circulation of air. In the Āyurvedic system these diseases are treated on the basis of air circulation. If from the beginning one takes care of the process of air circulation, such diseases cannot take place. From the Āyurveda as well as from the Śrīmad-Bhāgavatam it is clear that so many activities are going on internally and externally because of air alone, and as soon as there is some deficiency in the air circulation, these activities cannot take place. Here it is clearly stated, *netṛtvaṁ dravya-śabdayoḥ*. Our sense of proprietorship over action is also due to the activity of the air. If the air circulation is stifled, we cannot approach a place after hearing. If someone calls us, we hear the sound because of the air circulation, and we approach that sound or the place from which the sound comes. It is clearly said in this verse that these are all movements of the air. The ability to detect odors is also due to the action of the air.

(Śrīmad-Bhāgavatam 3.26.37, purport)

Śrīmad-Bhāgavatam... Veda means knowledge, I have several times explained. So Veda contains all kinds of knowledge. *Āyurveda*, the knowledge about medical science. *Dhanurveda*, the military science. *Āyurveda*, *Dhanurveda*, *Yajur veda*. Veda means knowledge.

(Lecture on Śrīmad-Bhāgavatam 1.9.49 Māyāpur, June 15, 1973)

But there is life after death. *tathā dehāntara prāptiḥ* (*Bg*. 2.13). There is life after death, simply change of body. Now, there are so many bodies — 8,400,000's of bodies. I can become a fly in my next life, according to my karma. Or I can become Brahmā in my next life. That is also according to karma. But there are varieties of life. So the so-called scientists, they do not know what is life after death, how it happens, how it is going on. This is a great science. That you can understand from the Vedic literature, not from your so-called scientific research. That is not possible.

So you feel the pulse and inquire the patient, Are you feeling like this? If he says, Yes, then it is confirmed. The disease is confirmed. Then the medicine is there. Very simple thing. Now in allopathic treatment, first of all you have to sacrifice one *chatak*(?) of blood, immediately. As soon as you go to the medical man, in your country, he will take so much blood. First of all you have to give your blood. Then fees. Then you have to purchase nonsense medicine. So here also there are nonsense *kavirājas* also. So unless one is expert in feeling the pulse, he is not *kavirāja*. That is the criterion.

*(Lecture on Śrīmad-*Bhāgavatam *1.10.6, Māyāpur, June 21, 1973)*

You should not eat the whole thing. You should eat half. And one fourth you shall fill up with water, and one fourth you should leave vacant so that there may be ventilation, your digestion will be easily done. This is Āyurvedic law. Even if you think that you can eat so much, you should not voluntarily eat so much. You should eat half, and one fourth you should fill up with water, and one fourth you should keep vacant for air ventilation. Then there will be no disease. It is hygienic principle. As soon as you eat more than what you can digest, you become diseased.

(Conversation, London, August 26, 1973)

Kapha, pitta, vāyu, known as the tri-dhātu, the three supports of the body. *Kapha* are the element that provide the structure for the body. *Pitta* are the elements that provide for the different kinds of digestion and transformation in the body. Vāta are the elements that allow movement of the different parts of the body. A kavirāja is an expert Āyurvedic doctor.

They have got their calculation: *kapha, pitta, vāyu. Tri-dhātu.* This body is a composition of these three *dhātus. yasyātma-buddhiḥ kuṇape tri-dhātuke* (*Bhag.* 10.84.13). *Kuṇape.* This is a bag created by the interaction of the three elements, namely, *kapha, pitta, vāyu*, or bile, mucus, and air. This is *kavirāja* treatment. They can understand the position of these three elements by feeling the pulse. This is Āyurvedic science. If one *kavirāja* can learn to feel the pulse, he can say everything. He can say when this man will die, today or tomorrow or... Accurately he will say. The pulse beating is so scientifically described in Āyurvedic science. As soon as he fixes up the pulse beating, immediately the formulas are there: Such kind of pulse beating will create such and such symptoms.

(Lecture on Śrīmad-Bhāgavatam 1.10.6, Māyāpur, June 21, 1973)

Prabhupāda: You have seen the birds, the sparrow, the crows. They are different birds. They have got different movements.
Tamāla Kṛṣṇa: Oh.
Prabhupāda: From the pulse beating, you study how it is beating.
Tamāla Kṛṣṇa: Like sparrow, like crow.
Prabhupāda: *Acchā.* Then, according to that, there is verse. Immediately everything will be arranged. The history. He will not ask, "Give me the history." He'll study the history from the pulse. That is *Āyurvedic*. So that is gone. To study *Āyurveda* is now lost. Nobody seriously takes *Āyurveda.*
Tamāla Kṛṣṇa: There is not much big money in it, I think.
Prabhupāda: Thing is allopathic is so popular now, nobody goes to *Āyurveda.*
Tamāla Kṛṣṇa: Yeah, there is no... You can't make a living very much.
Prabhupāda: They can give immediately, take. Although that is not very good, still, by lecture and by some strong medicine they can give him immediately. People like that. And Āyurveda is long term, and people cannot wait.

Tamāla Kṛṣṇa: Yeah. The cure is very slow.
Prabhupāda: And that is also not very sure, because the Āyurvedic physicians, they have not taken many cases. They cannot experience. Everything requires experience. These are the difficulties in *Āyurveda*. Still, some of the patent medicines, they are effective. Just like Cyavana-prāśa, Nava-yogendra, Yogendra-rasa. If they are properly prepared.

(Conversation, Bombay, April 5, 1977)

Harikeśa: How would the other necessities of life be taken care of, like medical things? If actually they have no knowledge, and they have to require to build these gigantic hospitals...
Prabhupāda: The *brāhmaṇas*, the *brāhmaṇas* will give you medical help. *Āyurveda*. They will read *Āyurveda*. They will give help.
Harikeśa: So the Āyurveda possibly can work nowadays.
Prabhupāda: Why not?
Harikeśa: Some people were telling me that the herbs had lost all their effectiveness in the Kali-yuga.
Prabhupāda: Then die. (laughter) Do you mean to say this modern medical treatment is guarantee for your living?
Harikeśa: No.
Prabhupāda: Then? That is also not guarantee. If you see the herbs and plants are no more effective, then if there is no guarantee in your modern medical, there is no guarantee. So why should you spend so much money? As soon as I go to a doctor, immediately twenty dollars. As soon as go to purchase some drugs, immediately twenty. If I have no money... And still that is not guarantee, so why shall I spend so much money?

(Morning Walk, Johannesburg, October 16, 1975)

Prabhupāda took Āyurvedic medicine. Once he said, "The three things that keep me healthy are my morning walk, my massage, and the Āyurvedic medicines." Every other morning he would take medicine made of freshly ground black cardamom seeds and a little pill of Yogendra-rasa, which was a heart medicine made of pearls and coral and other things. I would mix those two together and then add a quarter teaspoon of honey and mix that in with water. I ground and mixed the medicine with a pestle in a boat-shaped mortar, and Prabhupāda drank it out of that. One morning I had extra honey on the teaspoon, so I put it in the medicine. I thought,

"It'll be sweeter and maybe Prabhupāda will like it." He drank it, and about five minutes later he rang his bell. I came in, and he said, "How much honey did you put in the medicine?" I said, "I had a little extra on the spoon, about a half teaspoon." He said, "Keep it at a quarter. I'm intoxicated."

(Interview with Nanda Kumar Dāsa)

Śrīla Prabhupāda once said, "Did you ever notice that in old India, in the old remains of the architecture, that there are no hospitals? Why do you think that there were no hospitals." I said, "Well, less people were sick." He said, "They had sufficient money. They built wonderful temples out of stone and they also had Vedic knowledge, medical science. So the reason was that they were simply interested in cultivating Kṛṣṇa consciousness."

(Told by Tejiyas Dāsa)

Life to a Dead Body

The heavenly physicians like the Aśvinī-kumāras could give youthful life even to one who was advanced in age. Indeed, great yogis, with their mystic powers, can even bring a dead body back to life if the structure of the body is in order.

We have already discussed this in connection with Bali Mahārāja's soldiers and their treatment by Śukrācārya. Modern medical science has not yet discovered how to bring a dead body back to life or bring youthful energy to an old body, but from these verses we can understand that such treatment is possible if one is able to take knowledge from the Vedic information.

The Aśvinī-kumāras were expert in Āyurveda, as was Dhanvantari. In every department of material science, there is a perfection to be achieved, and to achieve it one must consult the Vedic literature. The highest perfection is to become a devotee of the Lord. To attain this perfection, one must consult Śrīmad-Bhāgavatam, which is understood to be the ripe fruit of the Vedic desire tree (*nigama-kalpa-taror galitaṁ phalaṁ*). *[Śrīmad-Bhāgavatam 1.1.3]*

(Śrīmad-Bhāgavatam 9.3.11, purport)

Āyurveda and Brahmins

Kapha, pitta, and vāyu. Kapha is mucus; *pitta*, bile; and *vāyu*, air. These things are being manufactured. After eating, these three things are being manufactured, and if they are well adjusted, parallel, then the body is healthy, and if there is more or less an imbalance, then there is disease. We have the Āyurveda — *ayur* means span of life, and Veda means knowledge.

The Vedic knowledge of the span of life is very simple. The doctors do not require a pathological laboratory, a clinic, no. They require to simply study these three elements, *kapha, pitta, vāyu*. Their science is to feel the pulse. You know, every one of you, that the pulse is moving: tick, tick, tick, tick. So they know the science of feeling the beating of the pulse. By this they understand the position of these three elements, *kapha, pitta, vāyu*. And by that position, they diagnose. In the Āyurveda there are symptoms: the veins are moving like this, the heart is moving like that, then the position is this. As soon as they understand the position, they verify the symptoms. They enquire from the patient, Do you feel like this? Do you feel like this? If he says, Yes, then it is confirmed. They feel how the pulse is beating, and the symptoms are confirmed; then the medicine is readied.

Immediately take the medicine. Formerly every *brāhmaṇa* used to learn these two sciences, Āyurveda and Jyotirveda, astrology, because the *kṣatriyas*, the *vaiśyās*, and the *Śūdras* needed the *brāhmaṇas*' advice for health and the future.

Everyone is inquisitive to learn the future, and everyone is concerned with health. So the *brāhmaṇas* would simply advise about health and the future. That was their profession, and people gave them eatables and cloth, so that they had nothing to do with working. Anyway, this body is a bag of the three elements, *yasyātma-buddhiḥ kuṇape tri-dhātuke* (*Śrīmad-Bhāgavatam* 10.84.13). The Bhāgavatam says, I am not this body. This is a vehicle. Just like we ride on a car; so I am not the car. Similarly, this is a *yantra*, a car. Kṛṣṇa, or God, has given me this car; I wanted it. That is stated in the *Bhagavad-gītā*: *Īśvaraḥ sarva-bhūtānāṁ hṛd-deśe 'rjuna tiṣṭhati* (*Bhagavad- gītā* 18.61). My dear Arjuna, the Lord as *paramātmā* is sitting in everyone's heart, *bhrāmayan sarva-bhūtāni yantrārūḍhāni māyayā*, and He is giving a chance to the living entity to travel, to wander,

sarva-bhūtāni, all over the universe. I am a soul. I have been given a nice car — it is not a nice car, but as soon as we get a car, however rotten it may be, we think that it is very nice [laughter] and identify with that car. I have got this car, I have got that car. One forgets, if one drives a very costly car, that he is a poor man. He thinks I am this car. This is bodily identification.
(Lecture on Śrīmad-Bhāgavatam 1.2.6, New Vrindavan, September 5, 1972)

You Are What You Eat

Prabhupāda: Yes, eating flesh sumptuously and get fat. Flesh-eaters get fatty very quickly, flesh-eaters. *Māṁsa.* The skin becomes increased for flesh-eating. You see in your country, the Russia? Russian beauty – big belly, fat. That...
Yamunā: Germans are like that too. Germans.
Prabhupāda: Germans. If you eat meat, you very quickly can get fat. Also too much ghee also. That is also. But ghee will increase your belly only. Just the Marwaris... (laughter) But by eating flesh you'll get sturdy, good lump of muscles. That is... In Āyurveda there is a chapter which is called *Dravya-guṇa.* There is a book, *Dravya-guṇa.* So they have analyzed so many different kinds of flesh – birds, beasts, animals. How they have analyzed? That if you eat this kind flesh you will get this kind of result. Hundreds of fleshes. What do they know? They can eat only cow's flesh or dog's flesh or hog's flesh. Yes. But there are so many, even birds, beasts, animals, and so many, analysis.
(Conversation, Indore, December 13, 1970)

Mr. Faill: There is none. To change the subject a little, is it necessary to follow certain eating habits to practice spiritual life?
Śrīla Prabhupāda: Yes, the whole process is meant to purify us, and eating is part of that purification. I think you have a saying, "You are what you eat," and that's a fact. Our bodily constitution and mental atmosphere are determined according to how and what we eat. Therefore the *Śāstras* recommend that to become Kṛṣṇa conscious, you should eat remnants of food left by Kṛṣṇa. If a tuberculosis patient eats something and you eat the remnants, you will be infected with tuberculosis. Similarly, if you eat *kṛṣṇa-prasādam,* then you will be infected with Kṛṣṇa consciousness. Thus our

process is that we don't eat anything immediately. First we offer the food to Kṛṣṇa, then we eat it. This helps us advance in Kṛṣṇa consciousness.

Mr. Faill: You are all vegetarians?

Śrīla Prabhupāda: Yes, because Kṛṣṇa is a vegetarian. Kṛṣṇa can eat anything because He is God, but in the *Bhagavad-gītā* (9.26) He says, "If one offers Me with love and devotion a leaf, a flower, fruit, or water, I will accept it." He never says, "Give Me meat and wine."

Mr. Faill: How about the tobacco question?

Śrīla Prabhupāda: Tobacco is also an intoxicant. We are already intoxicated by being in the bodily conception of life, and if we increase the intoxication, then we are lost.

Mr. Faill: You mean things like meat, alcohol, and tobacco just reinforce bodily consciousness?

Śrīla Prabhupāda: Yes. Suppose you have a disease and you want to be cured. You have to follow the instructions of a physician. if he says, "Don't eat this; eat only this," you have to follow his prescription. Similarly, we also have a prescription for being cured of the bodily conception of life: chanting Hare Kṛṣṇa, hearing about Kṛṣṇa's activities, and eating *kṛṣṇa-prasādam*. This treatment is the process of Kṛṣṇa consciousness.

(Science Self Realization Chap. 5)

Tamāla Kṛṣṇa: "As will be explained in the following verse, by performance of *yajñas*, the eatables become sanctified, and by eating sanctified foodstuffs one's very existence becomes purified."

Prabhupāda: Yes. Even George Bernard Shaw he has written, "You are what you eat." Your body is purified or unpurified according to the foodstuff you eat. Therefore we forbid, "Don't eat this, don't eat that." You have got sufficient food, grains, milk, butter, and fruits, sufficient. Why should you eat meat? That is not sanctified. But this is nature's product, offered to Kṛṣṇa, and you eat, and you become healthy and sanctified in mind, in body. Then you can understand Kṛṣṇa consciousness. You can make progress in that way. If your body is not sanctified, if it is impure, how can you understand the pure consciousness, or Kṛṣṇa consciousness? Therefore we have to follow these principles, regulations.

(Lecture on Bhagavad-gītā 3.11–19, Los Angeles, December 27, 1968)

Astrology and Āyurveda

Brahmānanda: To confirm the symptoms.
Prabhupāda: Yes. Confirm the symptoms. If he says: Yes, then immediately diagnosis is there. And as soon as diagnosis is there, the medicine is there. Simple method. Similarly, astrologers, they will see the constellation of the stars, and then the formula is there. If this star is now with this star, if that planet is with that planet, then this is the result. So this Āyurvedic astrologer and physician requires little clear brain. Otherwise, very nice. The research work is already there.

(Conversation Los Angeles, April 25, 1973)

Fire of Digestion

Dyotanam, illumination; *pacanam*, digesting; *pānam*, increasing thirst. If you don't feel thirsty, that means the *agni*, or the fire element within the stomach, is not working. *Agni-māndya*. *Māndya*, the word comes from *manda*. *Manda* means slow. So the Āyurvedic treatment, they say it, *agni-māndya*. So when there is *agni-māndya*, there is medicine how to ignite the fire again. There is fire within the stomach, within the abdomen.

*(Lecture on Śrīmad-*Bhāgavatam *3.26.40, Bombay, January 15, 1975)*

I am the fire of digestion in the bodies of all living entities, and I join with the air of life, outgoing and incoming, to digest the four kinds of foodstuff.

(Bhagavad-gītā 15.14)

According to Āyurvedic *Śāstra* [scripture], we understand that there is a fire in the stomach which digests all food sent there. When the fire is not blazing there is no hunger, and when the fire is in order we become hungry. Sometimes when the fire is not going nicely, treatment is required. In any case, this fire is representative of the Supreme Personality of Godhead. Vedic mantras (*Bṛhad-āraṇyaka Upaniṣad* 5.9.1) also confirm that the Supreme Lord or Brahman is situated in the form of fire within the stomach and is digesting all kinds of foodstuff (*ayam agnir vaiśvānaro yo 'yam antaḥ puruṣe yenedam annaṁ pacyate*). Therefore since He is helping the digestion of all kinds of foodstuff, the living entity is not independent in the eating process. Unless the Supreme Lord helps him in digesting, there is no possibility of eating. He thus produces and digests foodstuff, and by His grace we are enjoying life. In the *Vedanta-sutra* (1.2.27) this is also confirmed. *Śabdādibhyo 'ntaḥ pratiṣṭhānāc ca*: the Lord is situated within sound and within the body, within the air and even within the stomach as the digestive force. There are four kinds of foodstuff – some are swallowed, some are chewed, some are licked up, and some are sucked – and He is the digestive force for all of them.

(Bhagavad-gītā 15.14, purport)

Homeopathic Medicine

You have expressed the desire to become an Āyurvedic physician but I do not think that this proposal is very good. This science is not so important to us now because in your country there is ample facility for receiving medicines. Besides many of the herbs which are needed for Āyurvedic treatment would have to be sent here from India, and this is not very practical. This homeopathic medicine you have mentioned is not genuine and therefore is a bluff. So the first medicine which you should be concerned with is to chant Hare Kṛṣṇa and to become increasingly steady in Kṛṣṇa Consciousness.

(Letter to Upendra Dāsa, January 6, 1969)

And here... Just like homeopathics. They advertise, American homeopathics. But there is not a single shop of homeopathic medicine in America, not a single shop. And this is going on. All these bogus homeopathic practitioners, they write, American homeopathic medicine, and so on, so on. They do not allow this homeopathic medicine as bona fide practice. They are not so foolish that you will give water and it will be accepted as medicine. There you cannot ask even any medicine directly from the drug shop without doctor's prescription. If you go, offering to a medical drug shop, and give me this medicine, no, he'll not do so. Bring doctor's prescription. That is law.

*(Lecture on Śrīmad-*Bhāgavatam *6.1.22, Indore, December 13, 1970)*

No other engagement. Simply Kṛṣṇa. That is pure devotional service. But that is very difficult to achieve. People will not accept the simple thing. You give them big, big formulas, yoga system, *aṣṭāṅga-yoga*, they'll like it: It is something. Just like in homeopathic medicine, because it has no taste, there is no trouble to drink, people do not believe in it. But if you give them some very bitter, pungent medicine, Oh, it is something. Similarly, if you give the simple process, as Caitanya Mahāprabhu has given us, *harer nāma harer nāma harer nāmaiva kevalam, kalau nāstyeva nāstyeva nāstyeva gatir anyathā* (the chanting of the holy names of Lord Kṛṣṇa is the only process of self-realization recommended in the present age that we are living in) [Cc. Ādi 17.21], they'll not take it very seriously.

(Lecture on The Nectar of Devotion, Vṛndävana,, November 3, 1972)

Bhagavān: ...too simple.
Prabhupāda: Yes. Therefore they do not take it. Just like homeopathic medicine. You know homeopathic medicine?
Bhagavān: Oh, homeopathic medicine.
Prabhupāda: Yes, simply water. So they do not like to take it. Actually, they do not want God. They want *māyā*. Otherwise, if anyone wants God, Kṛṣṇa, there is no difficulty. Kṛṣṇa says, *man-manā bhava mad-bhakto mad-yājī māṁ namaskuru, mām evaiṣyasi* [Bg. 18.65].

(Morning Walk, Paris, June 9, 1974)

Massage

I am very glad to receive your recent letter. I am also glad to inform you that I am improving my health by the Grace of Kṛṣṇa. I don't believe in medicine or doctors, but I am practically perceiving that the massaging is helping me beyond expectation. Today I have taken a shower bath by myself and I am reciting from Śrīmad-Bhāgavatam and am enjoying the seashore here in New Jersey. I believe that within a fortnight I shall recoup my health sufficiently and be able to start for San Francisco and meet you all there.

(Letter to Nandarāṇī Dāsī, June 9, 1967)

So far my health is concerned, Gaurasundara is keeping me quite fit by massaging and Govinda Dāsī is supplying me *upmā* (cereal made from farina and vegetables). Perhaps you have never tasted what is *upmā*. But if Jadurāṇī can prepare it I shall send the formula.

(Letter to Satsvarūpa Dāsa, San Francisco, December 30, 1967)

I received the plan of my house in Māyāpur from Bombay address. I do not approve of this plan just yet. I liked one plan which I saw in London. Where is that original plan? Then I can make comparison. There was supposed to be a lift from the ground floor to the first floor. Also, why the guest rooms are upstairs, above me. Guest rooms are alright, but they cannot be occupied while I am there. There is also the question of the kitchen. And moreover, if there is no sunshine it will not be very nice. Will sunshine be able to enter my room?...(there are over-hanging verandas)...and is there a place on the roof open to the sun for taking massage?

(Letter to Girirāja Dāsa, Honolulu, May 26, 1976)

Prabhupāda called for me at 9:30 a.m. to begin his massage. He wanted to have it early because the sun was shining on the veranda outside his room. Whenever possible and if not too hot, he enjoys having his massage while exposed to the health-giving rays of the sun. It was finished by 11:00 a.m., and after bathing, he sat on his *āsana* in his room. With his eyes closed he remained in an upright position for about forty-five minutes. Occasionally his lips moved as he silently chanted or said something. He appeared to be completely absorbed – I wondered, perhaps, in Goloka Vṛndāvana?

(Transcendental Diary, Vol. 1, Chap. 9, January 18, 1976)

Medicine

Doctors give medicine and they speak surety, but there is no surety, and when there is no surety why should we break our four principles? I don't think there is guarantee of surety by taking this medicine with animal products, but if there is surety, you can take. But is very doubtful. When I come there I shall see what is wrong.

(Letter to Govinda Dāsa, February 12, 1972)

If one remembers Viṣṇu always, even though one is disturbed by many bad elements, one can be protected without a doubt.

The *Āyurveda-Śāstra* recommends, *auṣadhi cintayet viṣṇum*: even while taking medicine, one should remember Viṣṇu, because the medicine is not all and all and Lord Viṣṇu is the real protector. The material world is full of danger (*padaṁ padaṁ yad vipadām*).

Therefore one must become a Vaiṣṇava and think of Viṣṇu constantly. This is made easier by the chanting of the Hare Kṛṣṇa *mahā-mantra* [great sound vibration for spiritual elevation in this age]. Therefore Śrī Caitanya Mahāprabhu has recommended, *kīrtanīyaḥ sadā hariḥ* [always chant the names of God] [Cc. Ādi 17.31]

(*Śrīmad-Bhāgavatam 10.6.27–29, purport*)

Rāmeśvara: Do you think that they will adopt Indian medicine over Western medicine, things like that? Because there has to be some *varṇāśrama*.
Prabhupāda: No, medicine, if it is actually medicine, it will be accepted. It doesn't matter whether it is Indian or Western. If it is medicine it will be accepted.
Rāmeśvara: So that kind of research is in the mode of goodness.
Prabhupāda: That is already there. We have to make little research. It is already there. There are books, Āyurvedic books. They are very nice. Everything can be done. Dhanvantari. It is given by Dhanvantari *avatāra*, incarnation of Kṛṣṇa.
Rāmeśvara: You have written in the First Canto that we welcome scientists, doctors...
Prabhupāda: Yes, if it is beneficial.

(*Conversation, Bhuvaneśvara, January 21, 1977*)

Dr. Bhagat examined Śrīla Prabhupāda, diagnosing very high blood pressure and a weak heart. He said the uremia problem, which makes Prabhupāda's hands and feet swell, meant that his body produces too much water, and was probably the result of a kidney stone. He prescribed five different kinds of medicines: Lasix, a diuretic to eliminate excess water to be taken once a day with breakfast, Keflex, an antibiotic for the kidney infection to be ingested four times a day, Parafon Forte, a pain reliever, Valium, a psychotropic relaxant, and a sleeping pill. He also advised Prabhupāda not to take any salt or sugar.

Prabhupāda allowed us to purchase the medicines, but I have strong doubts that he will take them. And I know that he will never agree to a diet of no salt. He always insists that there must be some taste to his *prasādam*, otherwise he won't eat it.

(*Transcendental Diary, Vol. 3, Chap. 3, July 16, 1976*)

Although Dr. Patel knew very well His Divine Grace's opinion on taking medicine, he still tried some friendly persuasion and this led into a short discussion about Indian medicines. Dr. Patel said that there is a research plant in Calcutta that is extracting penicillin from cow dung.

Prabhupāda knew about it, adding that Dr. Monmohan Ghosh, a pathologist of Dr. Jagadisha Chandra Bose, conducted the original research proving the antiseptic properties of *gobar* (cow dung).

Dr. Patel said there were many medicinal properties in cow urine also. "*Go mūtra*, sir, there are so many hormones coming, and a big sample of hormones which can be resynthesized as human hormones."

Prabhupāda agreed, saying that if drunk, it was a good medicine for liver disease.

Dr. Patel expressed his concern again for Śrīla Prabhupāda's own health. Taking permission to raise his question he asked, "Now then, Arjuna was so advised that he should fight out. So in that case, I mean we all consider he was right to follow Kṛṣṇa's advice? Then if a man is overtaken by disease and if he fights out that ..."

Prabhupāda smiled at his persistence. "No, no, I don't say that he should not fight. It is my personal choice. Not that one should not take care of the body or one should not eat medicine, that is not ... I like this, 'Let me do without medicine.' That is my personal ..."

"What is medicine?" Dr. Patel asked. "Any herb is a medicine. Even food is a medicine."

"Whatever it may be," Prabhupāda said. "I don't decry medicine. That is not my business."

"No, no, I don't say decry. But you don't want to take advantage of medicine," Dr. Patel insisted.

"Medicine," Prabhupāda said objectively. "Just like a type of *vairāgya*, sometimes they do not eat. That does not mean eating is forbidden. It is not. It is my personal, I am trying to avoid, that's all.

"You have heard the name W. C. Bannerji? He was a big barrister. He was one of the three inaugurators of Congress in the beginning. So he had his friend, contemporary, he was a *brāhmaṇa*. He was taking daily his bath in the Ganges, and if he was diseased, was drinking Ganges water. So he became seriously sick. So this W. C. Bannerji, he was a big man. So he asked his permission to bring some doctor. 'You'll die in this way.' So he persisted, 'No, I shall simply drink this Ganges water.' So it is not that medical science is in defeated position."

(Transcendental Diary, Vol. 4, Chap. 2, August 15, 1976)

Nature Cure

"The Nature Cure Hospital as you have described it is all right."

(Letter to Mahāṁsa Swami, September 9, 1975)

Pilly Consciousness

Melbourne, 1974
Prabhupāda received another letter containing a report on the New York temple. The report stated that the devotees were regularly taking vitamin pills because they felt weak. Prabhupāda laughed, calling it "not Kṛṣṇa consciousness, but pilly consciousness."

"Wheat chaff and other unusable items are packed into vitamin pills and sold at high prices. There is a health fad," he explained, "and others are taking advantage and making money. This is going on." He then explained the source of vitamins: Just as cows eat grass and chaff and produce milk, vitamins were similarly coming from the fire of digestion."

(My Glorious Master, p. 235)

Surgery

As for your eye trouble, you need not take to an operation for your sickness. Doctors are not the Ultimate healer. This is Kṛṣṇa's position. In your Western countries, the doctors are very much fond of surgical operations. When there is no other alternative, of course we have to take shelter of such demoniac treatment, but as far as possible try to avoid that, and depend on Kṛṣṇa.

(Letter to Kṛṣṇa Dāsa, April 3, 1969)

Regarding this matter with your child, I cannot say, but at least I would not have agreed that the doctors perform this operation. In New York in 1968 when I was in the hospital they tried to operate my brain, but I left the hospital tactfully. Therefore I say that you never call a doctor for me or send me to the hospital. So it is up to you, but I would have not agreed.

(Letter to Māyāpurusasa Dāsa, November 4, 1975)

Prabhupāda: ...my Guru Mahārāja was in his last days, these rascal doctors injected... Our, this Kuñjabihārī, Tīrtha Mahārāja brought so many big, big doctors. And he protested, "Why are you giving me injection?" He protested. He personally said, "Why are you giving me injection? And if you bring a doctor, the rascals will not stop." Oh, that is our treatment. We must try our best." They will plead like that. "To give more trouble to the patient, that is our business." Inventing new medicines means inventing new means of giving trouble. That's all. As soon as you ask them whether by injection the life is guaranteed, they will say, "No. There is no guarantee. Let us try, make experiment." Yes. In hospital, as soon as you get...Whatever nonsense knowledge they have got, they make experiment, at the risk of other's life.

Haṁsadūta: When Himavatī broke her leg they wanted to operate. I said, "Oh, no, no chance. No operation." Then they immediately said, "Then maybe she'll never walk again."

Prabhupāda: Just see.

Haṁsadūta: So I said, "Well, how can we tell? They said, well, there's no way to tell." I said, "Suppose we operate. Then it's guaranteed that everything will be all right?" They said, "No." But they thought they should do that.

Prabhupāda: Yes. They canvass, they convince like that and make experiment. That is their business. They have no, I mean to say, assured idea. Simply experiment. All these hospitals, they are meant for making experiment. I think I have told you one story of my servant. Did I? Huh?

Haṁsadūta: No. Please tell us the story. (laughter)

Prabhupāda: (laughs) The servant was crying, "Oh! I am dying, I am dying, I am dying." So I immediately called ambulance and took her to the hospital. Then, when I went there, there were so many neophyte doctors. They experimented, and they said, "Immediate operation is required." "Why?" They gave us some technical terms. Then their leader doctor came. He said, "All right. Let us see this night. Then, next morning, we shall operate." So I asked him, "I can go? He may remain in your charge?" Yes. So I went, came back. And when I was absent, another servant of the neighbor, he told to my wife, that "*Babuji*..." *Babuji* means master. ...it is unnecessarily he has taken to hospital. He was drunk, and he was crying like that. (laughter) He drank." So my wife told that he was drunk, and he was therefore crying like that. "No, no. Doctor says that it is a serious case (laughter) and it is to be operated." And the next morning the servant came back. "And why you come back? You were to be operated?" "Oh, *thikhai*. It is now all right." Just see. The rascals were going to operate. He was drunk. In drunken state he was crying, and they took it a case of operation. That is my practical experience. Everything you take there: "Operation."

Devotee (1): That's a symptom of the modern civilization, Śrīla Prabhupāda.

Prabhupāda: Operation. That is... Demons are to be cheated like that. Simply operation. Simply operation. *Bas*.

Devotee (2): Also they're trying to get money.

Prabhupāda: Yes. Injection and operation. That is in their hands.

Tamāla Kṛṣṇa: Should we try to avoid getting injections as much as possible?

Prabhupāda: That is my opinion. But as soon as you go to a medical man, especially in your country, first of all, you have to give blood, immediately. (laughter) One ounce of blood immediately. First business. And then other injection. Because I underwent so many medical examination, I have got experience. For my immigration. I think, three or four times I was under health examination, and blood-taking, and injection. Of course, it is not very painful. That arrangement is there. But the business is like that, "First of all give your blood; then talk of other things." Better to die without a doctor. (laughter) That's the best principle. Don't call any doctor. Simply chant Hare Kṛṣṇa and die peacefully.

Tamāla Kṛṣṇa: But what about when you're not going to die... What about when you have some problems that's not fatal. Then who would we call?

Prabhupāda: Then go take injection. What can be done? (laughter) There is no alternative.

Devotee (1): How long will you be feeling bad from the injection?

Prabhupāda: If it remains simply for a while that is sufficient to kill you. There is no question of how long.

Devotee (1): It's just that you don't look very... You don't look like your normal self. There's no...

Prabhupāda: Sometimes they do business, simply water they inject. Yes. Simply water and take fee. They know there is no necessity of medicine; still, they will inject some water, distilled water, and take the fees. I have seen the doctors and some, "I mean to say, ordinary man, illiterate." What kind of treatment you want? Injection or medicine? "So naturally, he will say, The best one. I want to..." "Then you have to take injection."
Tamāla Kṛṣṇa: Or both. You might get both.
Prabhupāda: Yes. I have seen, they have spoken like that. Because the patient will think, "Oh, I take injection, I'll be very quickly cured." He will canvass like that. Because if he gives a bottle of medicine, that will not be very costly. But injection in his hand, he'll (have) at least five rupees, that much. So he'll canvass like that, "What kind of treatment you want, injection or ordinary medicine." So he'll say, "Sir, best medicine I want." "Then you take injection." That's all. It is a fact that the whole human civilization is a society of cheaters and cheated. That's all. Any field. *Māyāiva vyavaharite*. The whole world in this *Kali-yuga*: *māyāiva vyavaharite*. *Vyavaharite* means ordinary dealings, there will be cheating. Ordinarily, there will be cheating. Daily affairs. Not to speak of very great things. Ordinary dealings, there will be cheating. That is stated in the *Bhāgavata* (*Śrīmad*-Bhāgavatam), *māyāiva vyavahari*. The sooner you get out of this scene is better. That is Kṛṣṇa consciousness. So long you live, you simply chant Hare Kṛṣṇa and preach Kṛṣṇa's glories, and that's all. Otherwise, you should know that this is a dangerous place. *Padaṁ padaṁ yad vipadāṁ*. In every step there is danger.

(Conversation, Gorakhpur, February 14, 1971)

Vaccines

Brahmānanda: Actually, when I was in Germany, there was evidence of how the scientists increased disease. They invented some vaccine to counteract influenza, and they injected all of Germany with this vaccine. But what happened was sometimes the body builds up resistance to these vaccines and produces another germ. So, as a result, another type of influenza was created, which was far more worse than the previous. It made people get fever for four and five days straight, 105 degrees.
Prabhupāda: That is the way of... They have discovered this streptomycin, for tuberculosis, that if one takes too many injections of streptomycin,

then it does not act.
Devotee: He becomes immune.
Prabhupāda: Yes.
Brahmānanda: So as a result of the vaccine they created a worse type of influenza, and they have nothing to counteract that worse type. So now they have to invent another type.
Prabhupāda: These rascals give trouble to the people, especially in India. They are not after the vaccine. They will catch people and force them. Just see. This is going on. (indistinct) others are avoiding, they are going, going this way, that way. Sometimes they fall, they do not know, and capture (indistinct). These rascals are creating havoc. Only to kick them on their face with shoes. That's all. The so-called scientists and biologists and... They do not know anything.

(Conversation, Hydrabad, April 14, 1975)

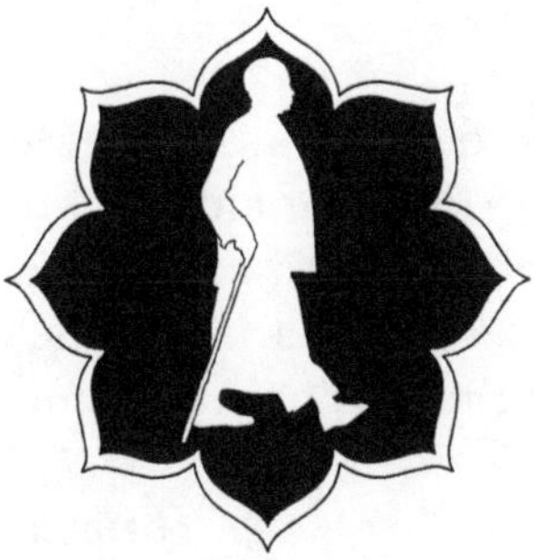

Chapter 5

Some Amazing Stories from the Scriptures

Hiraṇyakaśipu and Lord Brahmā

Hiraṇyakaśipu wanted to become immortal. He wanted not to be conquered by anyone, not to be attacked by old age and disease, and not to be harassed by any opponent. Thus he wanted to become the absolute ruler of the entire universe. With this desire, he entered the valley of Mandara Mountain and began practicing a severe type of austerity and meditation. Seeing Hiraṇyakaśipu engaged in this austerity, the demigods returned to their respective homes, but while Hiraṇyakaśipu was thus engaged, a kind of fire began blazing from his head, disturbing the entire universe and its inhabitants, including the birds, beasts and demigods. When all the higher and lower planets became too hot to live on, the demigods, being disturbed, left their abodes in the higher planets and went to see Lord Brahmā, praying to him that he curtail this unnecessary heat. The demigods disclosed to Lord Brahmā Hiraṇyakaśipu's ambition to become immortal, overcoming his short duration of life, and to be the master of all the planetary systems, even Dhruvaloka.

Upon hearing about the purpose of Hiraṇyakaśipu's austere meditation, Lord Brahmā, accompanied by the great sage Bhṛgu and great personalities like Dakṣa, went to see Hiraṇyakaśipu.

(Śrīmad-Bhāgavatam 7.3, Summary)

Lord Brahmā, who is carried by a swan airplane, at first could not see where Hiraṇyakaśipu was, for Hiraṇyakaśipu's body was covered by an anthill and by grass and bamboo sticks. Because Hiraṇyakaśipu had been there for a long time, the ants had devoured his skin, fat, flesh and blood. Then Lord Brahmā and the demigods spotted him, resembling a cloud – covered sun, heating all the world by his austerity. Struck with wonder, Lord Brahmā began to smile and then addressed him as follows.

(*Śrīmad-Bhāgavatam 7.3.15-16)*

The living entity can live merely by his own power, without the help of skin, marrow, bone, blood and so on, because it is said, *asaṅgo 'yaṁ puruṣaḥ* – the living entity has nothing to do with the material covering. Hiraṇyakaśipu performed a severe type of *tapasya*, austerity, for many long years. Indeed, it is said that he performed the *tapasya* for one hundred heavenly years. Since one day of the demigods equals six of our months, certainly this was a very long time. By nature's own way, his body had been almost consumed by earthworms, ants and other parasites, and therefore even Brahmā was at first unable to see him. Later, however, Brahmā could ascertain where Hiraṇyakaśipu was, and Brahmā was struck with wonder to see Hiraṇyakaśipu's extraordinary power to execute *tapasya*. Anyone would conclude that Hiraṇyakaśipu was dead because his body was covered in so many ways, but Lord Brahmā, the supreme living being in this universe, could understand that Hiraṇyakaśipu was alive but covered by material elements.

(*Śrīmad-Bhāgavatam 7.3.15–16, purport)*

I have been very much astonished to see your endurance. In spite of being eaten and bitten by all kinds of worms and ants, you are keeping your life air circulating within your bones. Certainly this is wonderful.

(*Śrīmad-Bhāgavatam 7.3.18)*

It appears that the soul can exist even through the bones, as shown by the personal example of Hiraṇyakaśipu. When great yogis are in *samādhi*, even when their bodies are buried and their skin, marrow, blood and so on have all been eaten, if only their bones remain they can exist in a transcendental position. Very recently an archaeologist published findings indicating that Lord Christ, after being buried, was exhumed and that he then went to Kashmir. There have been many actual examples of yogis' being buried in trance and exhumed alive and in good condition several hours later. A yogi can keep himself alive in a transcendental state even if buried not only for many days but for many years.

(Śrīmad-Bhāgavatam 7.3.18, purport)

Even saintly persons like Bhṛgu, born previously, could not perform such severe austerities, nor will anyone in the future be able to do so. Who within these three worlds can sustain his life without even drinking water for one hundred celestial years?

(Śrīmad-Bhāgavatam 7.3.19)

It appears that even if a yogi does not drink a drop of water, he can live for many, many years by the yogic process, though his outer body be eaten by ants and moths.

(Śrīmad-Bhāgavatam 7.3.19, purport)

Śrī Nārada Muni continued: After speaking these words to Hiraṇyakaśipu, Lord Brahmā, the original being of this universe, who is extremely powerful, sprinkled transcendental, infallible, spiritual water from his kamaṇḍalu (water pot) upon Hiraṇyakaśipu's body, which had been eaten away by ants and moths. Thus he enlivened Hiraṇyakaśipu.

(Śrīmad-Bhāgavatam 7.3.22)

Lord Brahmā is the first created being within this universe and is empowered by the Supreme Lord to create. *tene Brahmā hṛdā ya ādi-kavaye*: [SB 1.1.1] the *adi deva*, or *adi-kavi* – the first living creature – was personally taught by the Supreme Personality of Godhead through the heart. There was no one to teach him, but since the Lord is situated within Brahmā's heart, Brahmā was educated by the Lord Himself. Lord Brahmā, being especially empowered, is infallible in doing whatever he wants. This is the meaning of the word *amogha rādhasā*. He desired to restore Hiraṇyakaśipu's original body, and therefore, by sprinkling transcendental water from his waterpot, he immediately did so.

(Śrīmad-Bhāgavatam 7.3.22, purport)

As soon as he was sprinkled with the water from Lord Brahmā's water pot, Hiraṇyakaśipu arose, endowed with a full body with limbs so strong that they could bear the striking of a thunderbolt. With physical strength and a bodily luster resembling molten gold, he emerged from the anthill a completely young man, just as fire springs from fuel wood.

(Śrīmad-Bhāgavatam 7.3.23)

Hiraṇyakaśipu was revitalized, so much so that his body was quite competent to tolerate the striking of thunderbolts. He was now a young man with a strong body and a very beautiful bodily luster resembling molten gold. This is the rejuvenation that took place because of his severe austerity and penance.

(Śrīmad-Bhāgavatam 7.3.23, purport)

Indra and His Elephant

Seeing Vṛtrāsura's disposition, Indra, the King of heaven, became intolerant and threw at him one of his great clubs, which are extremely difficult to counteract. However, as the club flew toward him, Vṛtrāsura easily caught it with his left hand.

O King Parīkṣit, the powerful Vṛtrāsura, the enemy of King Indra, angrily struck the head of Indra's elephant with that club, making a tumultuous sound on the battlefield. For this heroic deed, the soldiers on both sides glorified him.

Struck with the club by Vṛtrāsura like a mountain struck by a thunderbolt, the elephant Airāvata, feeling great pain and spitting blood from its broken mouth, was pushed back fourteen yards. In great distress, the elephant fell, with Indra on its back.

When he saw Indra's carrier elephant thus fatigued and injured and when he saw Indra morose because his carrier had been harmed in that way, the great soul Vṛtrāsura, following religious principles, refrained from again striking Indra with the club. Taking this opportunity, Indra touched the elephant with his nectar-producing hand, thus relieving the animal's pain and curing its injuries. Then the elephant and Indra both stood silently.

(Śrīmad-Bhāgavatam 6.11.9–11)

Sanātana Gosvāmī and Itching Sores

Śrīla Sanātana Gosvāmī came alone from Mathurā to Jagannātha Purī to see Lord Caitanya. Because of bathing in bad water and not getting enough food every day while traveling on the path through Jharikhaṇḍa Forest, he developed a disease that made his body itch. Suffering greatly from this itching, he resolved that in the presence of Śrī Caitanya Mahāprabhu he would throw himself under the wheel of Jagannātha's car and in this way commit suicide...

One day Śrī Caitanya Mahāprabhu said to Sanātana Gosvāmī, "Your decision to commit suicide is the result of the mode of ignorance. One cannot get love of God simply by committing suicide. You have already dedicated your life and body to My service; therefore your body does not belong to you, nor do you have any right to commit suicide. I have to execute many devotional services through your body. I want you to preach the cult of devotional service and go to Vṛndāvana to excavate the lost holy places." After having thus spoken, Śrī Caitanya Mahāprabhu left, and Haridāsa Thākura and Sanātana Gosvāmī had many talks about this subject.

One day Sanātana Gosvāmī was summoned by Śrī Caitanya Mahāprabhu, who wanted him to come to Yameśvara-ṭoṭā. Sanātana Gosvāmī reached the Lord through the path along the beach by the sea. When Śrī Caitanya Mahāprabhu asked Sanātana Gosvāmī which way he had come, Sanātana replied, "Many servitors of Lord Jagannātha come and go on the path by the Siṁha-dvāra gate of the Jagannātha temple. Therefore, I did not go by that path, but instead went by the beach." Sanātana Gosvāmī did not realize that there were burning blisters on his feet because of the heat of the sand. Śrī Caitanya Mahāprabhu was pleased to hear about Sanātana Gosvāmī's great respect for the temple of Lord Śrī Jagannātha.

Because his disease produced wet sores on his body, Sanātana Gosvāmī used to avoid embracing Śrī Caitanya Mahāprabhu, but nevertheless the Lord would embrace him by force. This made Sanātana Gosvāmī very unhappy, and therefore he consulted Jagadānanda Paṇḍita about what he should do. Jagadānanda advised him to return to Vṛndāvana after the car festival of Jagannātha, but when Śrī Caitanya Mahāprabhu heard about this instruction,

He chastised Jagadānanda Paṇḍita and reminded him that Sanātana Gosvāmī was senior to him and also more learned. Śrī Caitanya Mahāprabhu informed Sanātana Gosvāmī that because Sanātana was a pure devotee, the Lord was never inconvenienced by his bodily condition. Because the Lord was a *sannyāsī*, He did not consider one body better than another. The Lord also informed him that He was maintaining Sanātana and the other devotees just like a father. Therefore the moisture oozing from Sanātana's itching skin did not affect the Lord at all. After speaking with Sanātana Gosvāmī in this way, the Lord again embraced him, and after this embrace, Sanātana Gosvāmī became free from the disease.

(Caitanya-caritamrta, Antya-lilā 4, Summary)

The Leper Vāsudeva and Lord Caitanya

There was also a *brāhmaṇa* named Vāsudeva, who was a great person but was suffering from leprosy. Indeed, his body was filled with living worms. Although suffering from leprosy, the *brāhmaṇa* Vāsudeva was enlightened. As soon as one worm fell from his body, he would pick it up and place it back again in the same location. Then one night Vāsudeva heard of Lord Caitanya Mahāprabhu's arrival, and in the morning he came to see the Lord at the house of Kūrma.

When the leper Vāsudeva came to Kūrma's house to see Caitanya Mahāprabhu, he was informed that the Lord had already left. The leper then fell to the ground unconscious. When Vāsudeva, the leper *brāhmaṇa*, was lamenting due to not being able to see Caitanya Mahāprabhu, the Lord immediately returned to that spot and embraced him. When Śrī Caitanya Mahāprabhu touched him, both the leprosy and his distress went to a distant place. Indeed, Vāsudeva's body became very beautiful, to his great happiness.

(Caitanya-caritāmṛta, Madhya-lila 7. 136–141)

Śrīvāsa Ṭhākura's Son Dies

This incident is described as follows by Śrīla Bhaktivinoda Ṭhākura in his *Amṛta-pravāha-bhāṣya*. One night while Śrī Caitanya Mahāprabhu was dancing with His devotees at the house of Śrīvāsa Ṭhākura, one of Śrīvāsa Ṭhākura's sons, who was suffering from some disease, died. Śrīvāsa Ṭhākura was so patient, however, that he did not allow anyone to express sorrow by crying, for he did not want the *kīrtana* going on at his house to be disturbed. Thus *kīrtana* continued without a sound of lamentation. But when the *kīrtana* was over, Caitanya Mahāprabhu, who could understand the incident, declared, "There must have been some calamity in this house." When He was then informed about the death of Śrīvāsa Ṭhākura's son, He expressed His regret, saying, "Why was this news not given to Me before?" He went to the place where the son was lying dead and asked him, "My dear boy, why are you leaving the house of Śrīvāsa Ṭhākura?" The dead son immediately replied, "I was living in this house as long as I was destined to live here. Now that the time is over, I am going elsewhere, according to Your direction. I am Your eternal servant, a dependent living being. I must act only according to Your desire. Beyond Your desire, I cannot do anything. I have no such power." Hearing these words of the dead son, all the members of Śrīvāsa Ṭhākura's family received transcendental knowledge. Thus there was no cause for lamentation. This transcendental knowledge is described in the *Bhagavad-gītā* (2.13): *tathā dehāntara-prāptir dhīras tatra na muhyati.* When someone dies, he accepts another body; therefore sober persons do not lament. After the discourse between the dead boy and Śrī Caitanya Mahāprabhu, funeral ceremonies were performed, and Lord Caitanya assured Śrīvāsa Ṭhākura, "You have lost one son, but Nityānanda Prabhu and I are your eternal sons. We shall never be able to give up your company." This is an instance of a transcendental relationship with Kṛṣṇa. We have eternal transcendental relationships with Kṛṣṇa as His servants, friends, fathers, sons or conjugal lovers. When the same relationships are pervertedly reflected in this material world, we have relationships as the sons, fathers, friends, lovers, masters or servants of others, but all these relationships are subject to termination within a definite period. If we revive our relationship with Kṛṣṇa, however, by the grace of Śrī Caitanya Mahāprabhu our eternal relationship will never break to cause our lamentation.

(Caitanya-caritamrta, Ādi-līlā 17.229, purport)

Sāraṅga Ṭhākura and Murāri Caitanya dāsa

Another name of Ṭhākura Sāraṅga dāsa was Śārṅga Ṭhākura. Sometimes he was also called Śārṅgapāṇi or Śārṅgadhara. He was a resident of Navadvīpa in the neighborhood known as Modadruma-dvīpa, and he used to worship the Supreme Lord in a secluded place on the bank of the Ganges. He was not accepting disciples, but he was repeatedly being inspired from within by the Supreme Personality of Godhead to do so. Thus one morning he decided, 'Whomever I see I shall make my disciple.' When he went to the bank of the Ganges to take his bath, by chance he saw a dead body floating in the water, and he touched it with his feet. This immediately brought the body to life, and Ṭhākura Sāraṅga dāsa accepted him as his disciple. This disciple later became famous as Ṭhākura Murāri, and his name is always associated with that of Śrī Sāraṅga.

(Caitanya-caritamrta, Ādi-lilā 10.113, purport)

Prahlāda Mahārāja Fed Poison

Hiraṇyakaśipu could not kill his son by throwing him beneath the feet of big elephants, throwing him among huge, fearful snakes, employing destructive spells, hurling him from the top of a hill, conjuring up illusory tricks, administering poison, starving him, exposing him to severe cold, winds, fire and water, or throwing heavy stones to crush him. When Hiraṇyakaśipu found that he could not in any way harm Prahlāda, who was completely sinless, he was in great anxiety about what to do next.

(Śrīmad-Bhāgavatam 7.5.43–44)

Cyavana Muni

When the heavenly physicians the Aśvinī-kumāra brothers once visited Cyavana Muni, the muni requested them to give him back his youth. These two physicians took Cyavana Muni to a particular lake, in which they bathed and regained full youth.

(Śrīmad-Bhāgavatam 9.3, Summary)

The Hunchback Kubja Becomes Beautiful

After leaving the florist's place, Kṛṣṇa and Balarāma saw a hunchbacked young woman carrying a dish of sandalwood pulp through the streets. Since Kṛṣṇa is the reservoir of all pleasure, He wanted to make all His companions joyous by cutting a joke with the hunchbacked woman. Kṛṣṇa addressed her, "O tall young woman, who are you? Tell Me, for whom are you carrying this sandalwood pulp in your hand? I think you should offer this sandalwood to Me, and if you do so I am sure you will be fortunate." Kṛṣṇa is the Supreme Personality of Godhead, and He knew everything about the hunchback. By His inquiry He indicated that there was no use in serving a demon; she would do better to serve Kṛṣṇa and Balarāma and get an immediate result of the service.

The woman replied to Kṛṣṇa, "My dear Śyāmasundara, dear beautiful dark boy, You may know that I am engaged as a maidservant of Kaṁsa. I am supplying him pulp of sandalwood daily. The King is very much pleased with me for supplying this nice thing, but now I see that there is no one who can better be served by this pulp of sandalwood than You two brothers." Being captivated by the beautiful features of Kṛṣṇa and Balarāma, Their talking, Their smiling, Their glancing and Their other activities, the hunchbacked woman began to smear all the pulp of sandalwood over Their bodies with great satisfaction and devotion. The two transcendental brothers, Kṛṣṇa and Balarāma, were naturally beautiful and had beautiful complexions, and They were nicely dressed in colorful garments. The upper portions of Their bodies were already very attractive, and when the hunchbacked woman smeared Their bodies with sandalwood pulp, They looked even more beautiful. Kṛṣṇa was very much pleased by this service, and He began to consider how to reward her. In other words, in order to draw the attention of the Lord, the Kṛṣṇa conscious devotee has to serve Him in great love and devotion. Kṛṣṇa cannot be pleased by any action other than transcendental loving service unto Him. Thinking like this, Lord Kṛṣṇa pressed the feet of the hunchbacked woman with His toes and, capturing her cheeks with His fingers, gave her a jerk in order to make her straight. At once the hunchbacked woman became a beautiful straight girl, with broad hips, thin waist and very nice, well-shaped breasts. Since Kṛṣṇa was pleased with the service of the hunchbacked woman, and since she was touched by Kṛṣṇa's hands, she became the most beautiful girl among women. This incident shows that by serving Kṛṣṇa the devotee immediately becomes elevated to the most exalted position in all respects. Devotional service is so potent that anyone who takes to it becomes qualified with all godly qualities. Kṛṣṇa was attracted to the hunchbacked woman not for her beauty but for her service; as soon as she rendered service, she immediately became the most beautiful woman. A Kṛṣṇa conscious person does not have to be qualified or beautiful; after becoming Kṛṣṇa conscious and rendering service unto Kṛṣṇa, he becomes very much qualified and beautiful.

(Kṛṣṇa: The Supreme Personality of Godhead, Chap. 42)

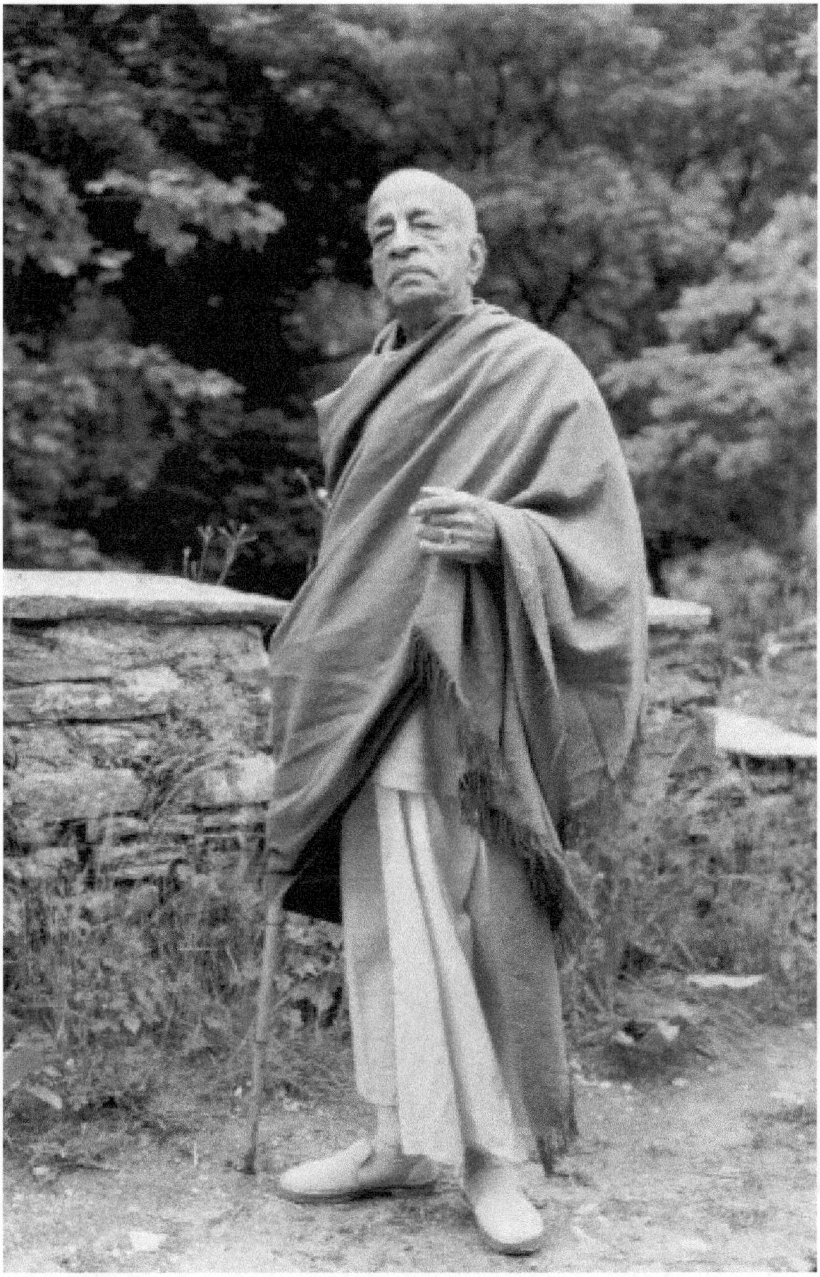

A.C. Bhaktivedanta Swami Prabhupada

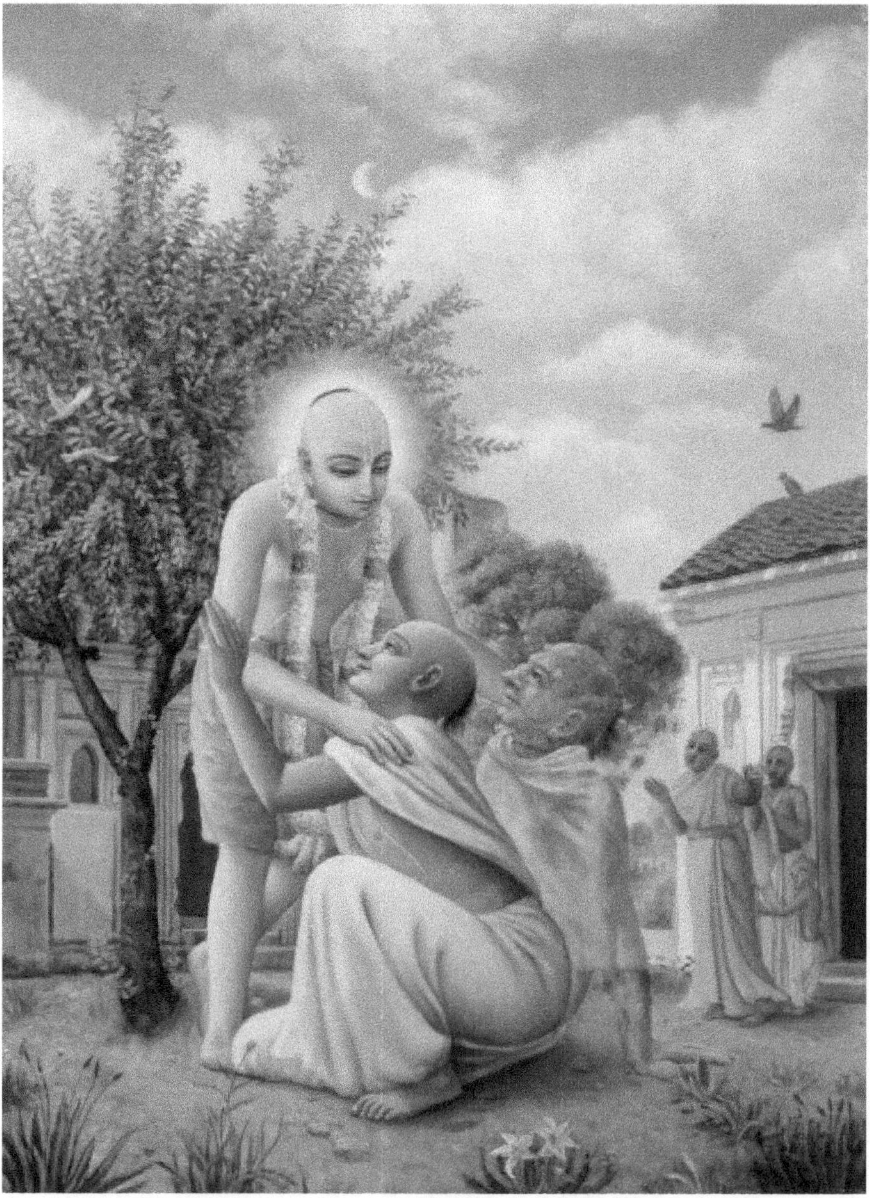

(1) Lord Caitanya's touch makes Vasudeva's leprosy disappear and his body become very beautiful.

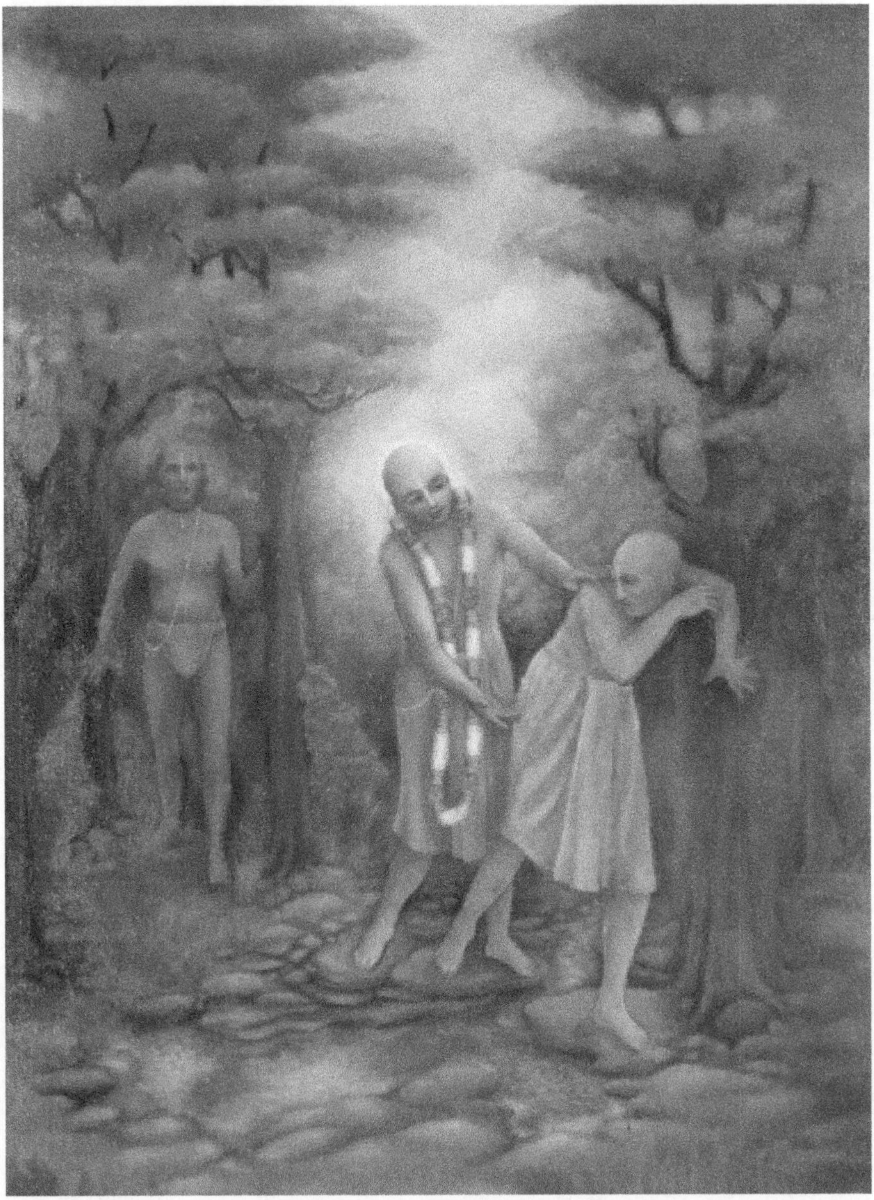

(2) Lord Caitanya cures Sanatana Goswami who suffered from itching sores all over his body.

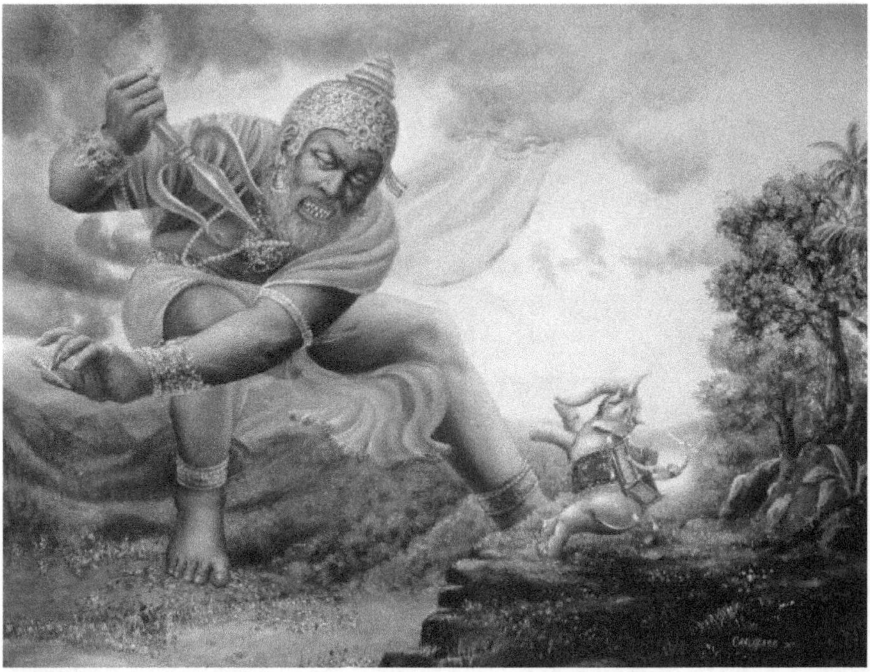

(3) Indra cures his wounded elephant with the touch of his hand.

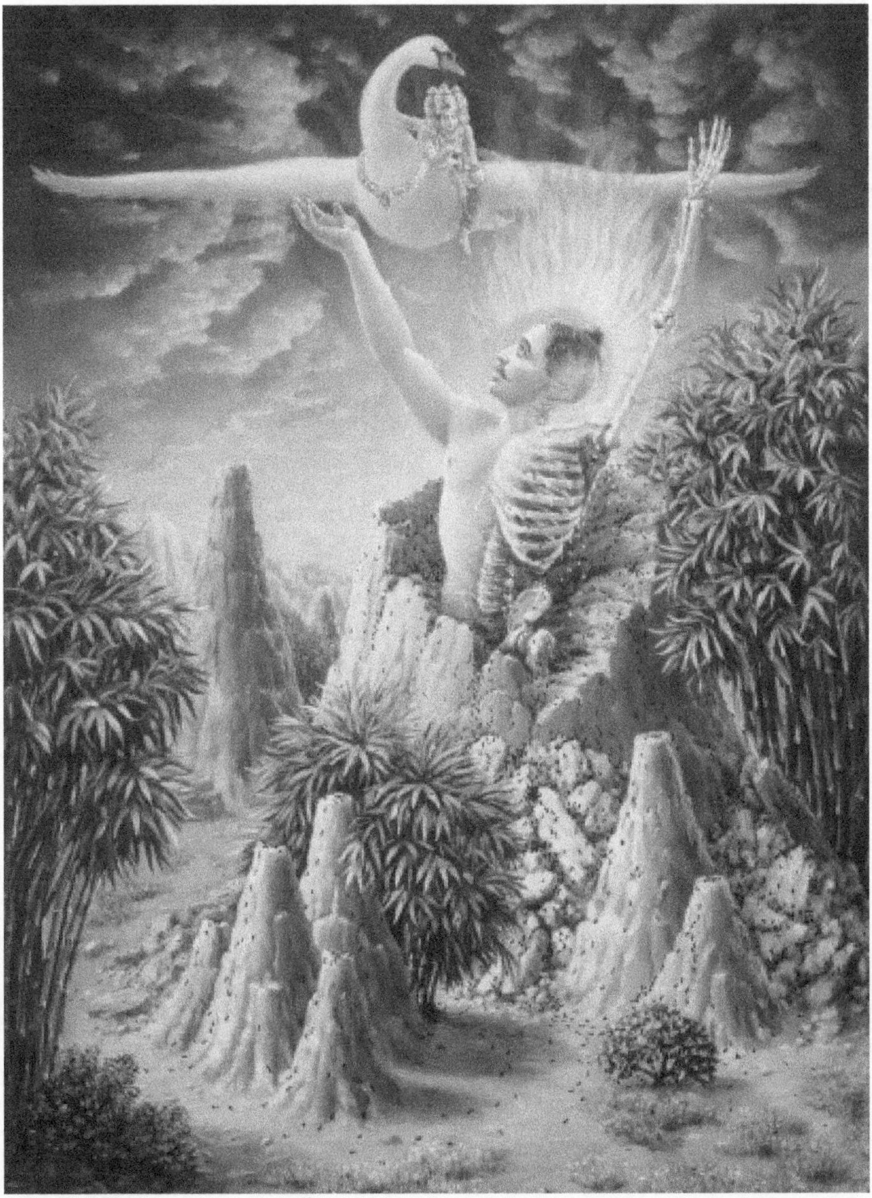

(4) *Lord Brahma revives Hiranyakasipu's body with full beauty and a golden luster.*

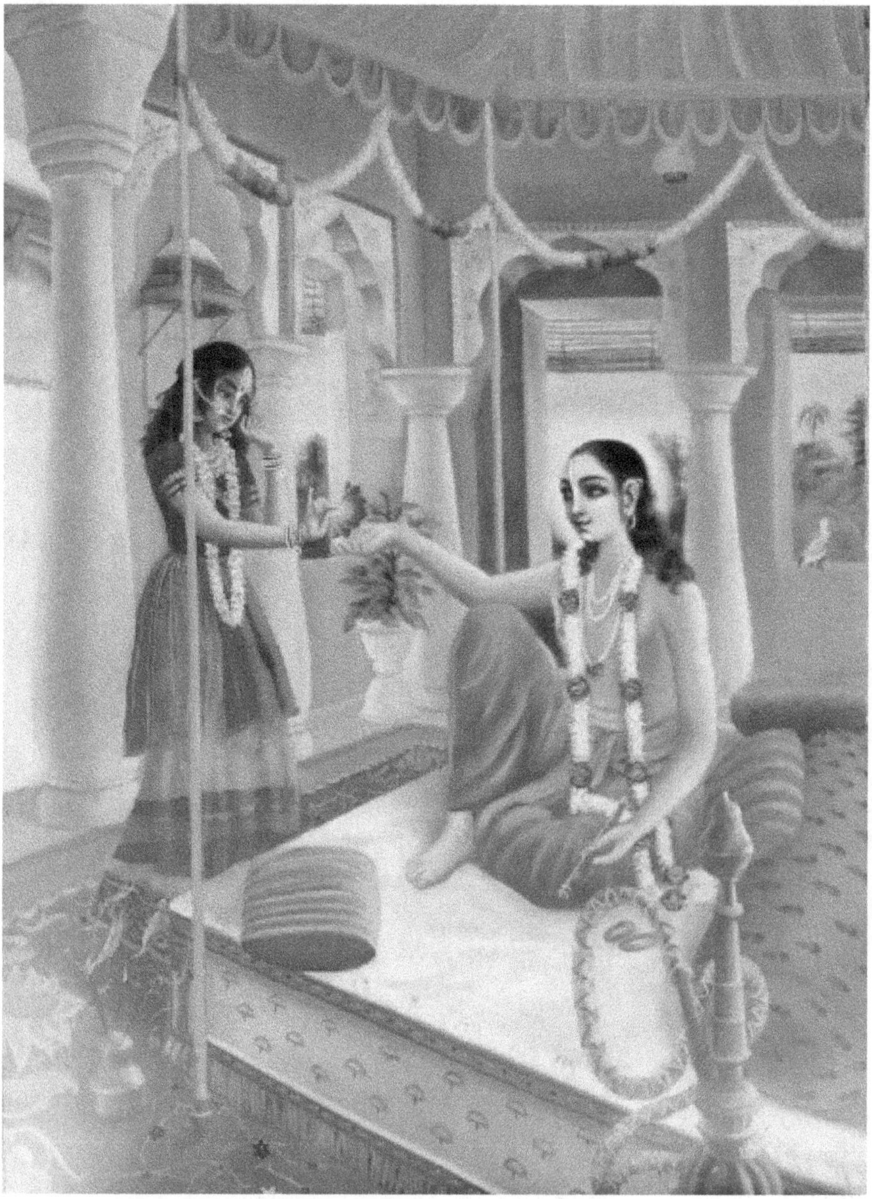

(5) Lord Krsna transforms the hunchback Kubja into a beautiful girl.

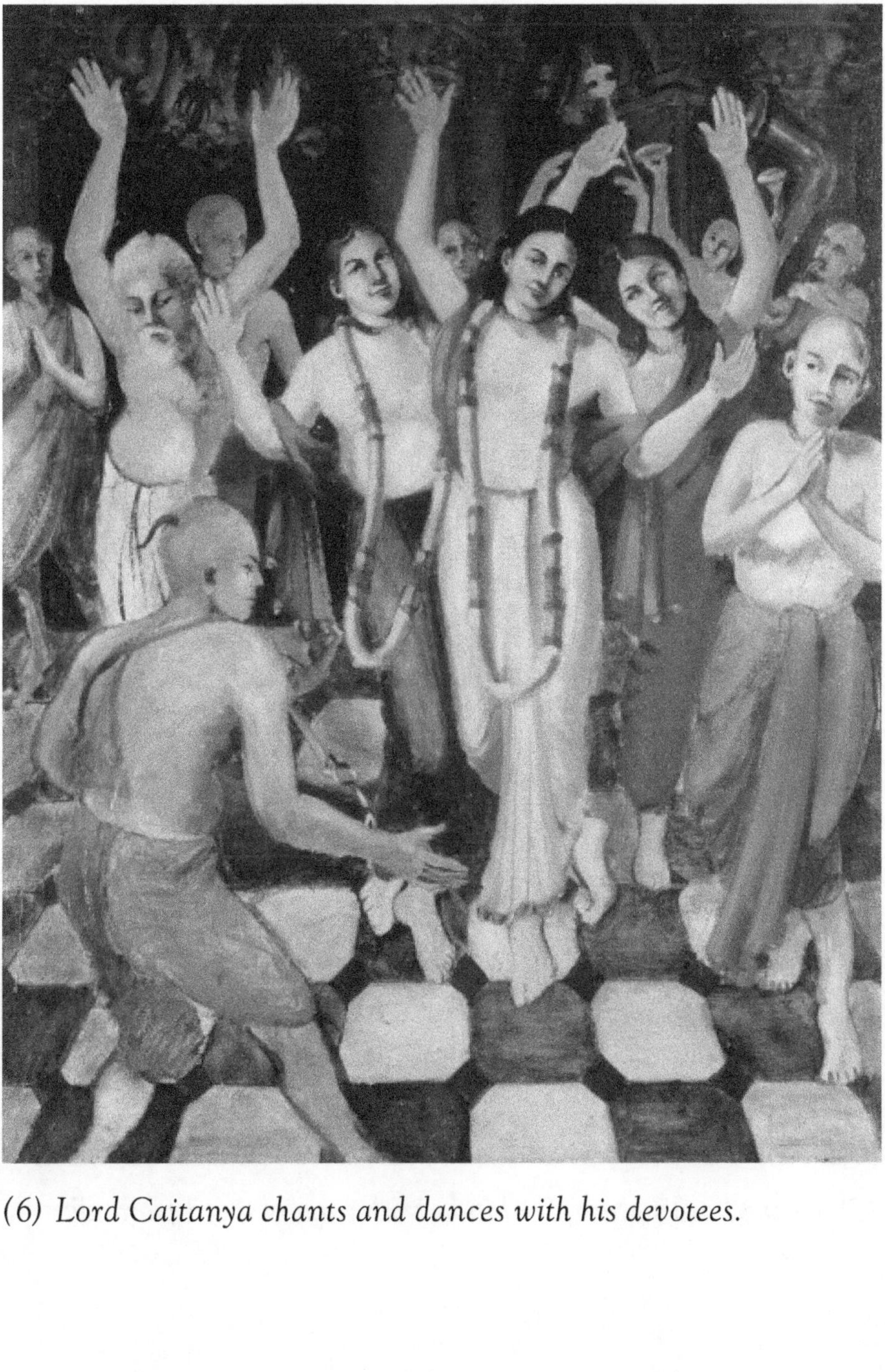

(6) Lord Caitanya chants and dances with his devotees.

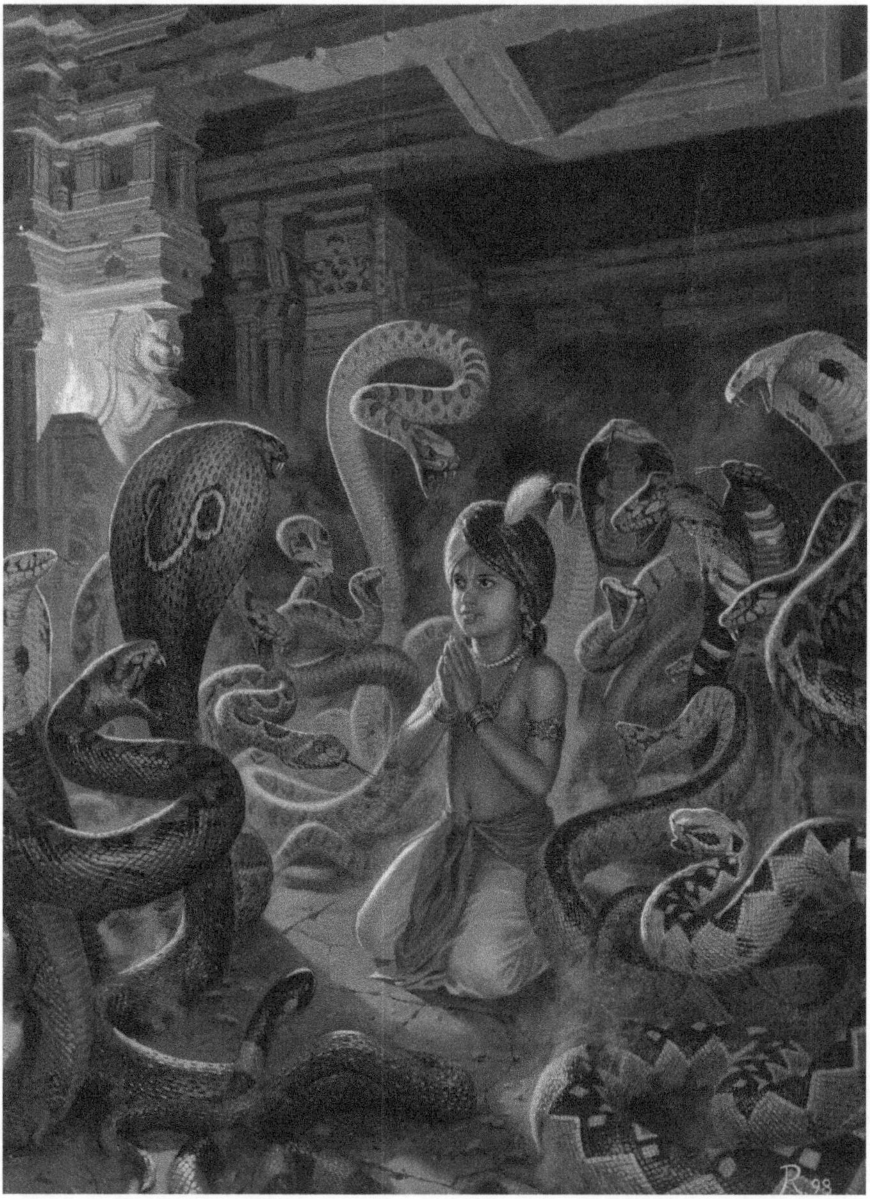

(7) By the Lord's grace, Prahlada Maharaja is saved from all harm.

Chapter 6
Articles on Health by Prahlādānanda Swami

Āyurveda 101

Āyurveda is the ancient science of life. "Āyur" in Sanskrit means "life" and "veda" means "knowledge" or "science." In this article, I will explain some of the basic principles of Āyurveda.

The science called Āyurveda deals with the five gross elements — Earth, Water, Fire, Air, and Ether — and three subtle elements — Mind, Intelligence, and False Ego. These eight elements constitute the material energy.

In general, when we speak of Earth with a capital "E", we refer to material elements that have the primary characteristic of being solid. Therefore, any substance made of clay, stone, metal, wood, or other "solid" matter would be classified as belonging to the Earth category. Those material substances that have liquidity as their primary characteristic belong to the category of Water. Fire refers to radiant or effulgent substances, and Air refers to those substances that move and have the power to move other things. Ether is the space in which other elements are contained.

The combination of different physical elements produces six different tastes: sweet, sour, salty, pungent, astringent, and bitter. Sweet taste is a combination of Water and Earth and has properties similar to those two elements. Because Earth is solid matter, sweet taste is the heaviest of all the tastes and most like *kapha*. It is found in its pure form in sugar. Sour is a combination of Earth and Fire and will help the digestion. It is found in its pure form in alcohol. Similarly, the salty taste, found in its pure form in salt, is a combination of Water and Fire, and when present in food in the proper proportion, it increases the taste of food. The pungent taste is a combination Fire and Air. As air can fan a fire, the pungent taste is the hottest of the tastes and is present in its pure form in chilies. Astringent is a combination of Earth and Air and causes the mouth to pucker when ingested. It is found in its pure form in the tannins of teas. Bitter is a combination of Air and Ether and is found in its pure form in bitter melon or neem leaves.

A soul receives a material body according to the physical state and the consciousness of the parents at the time of conception. This body is said to be of a certain *prakṛti* or combination of the above-mentioned material elements in what is called a "*doṣa*." For instance, the combination of Earth and Water together in the body is called "*kapha dosha*." In a healthy material body, Earth and Water exist together in a balanced state, but when there is a lack of balance between these two elements problems arise. Too much Earth and not enough Water can produce diseases such as kidney or gall bladder stones. Too much Water and not enough Earth can produce edema (an abnormal accumulation of fluid beneath the skin, or in one or more cavities of the body).

In a similar way, Water and Fire combine together in a physical body. When there is an imbalance of too much Water and not enough Fire, indigestion results. Too much Fire and not enough Water results in ulcers. Air and Ether must also be in harmony to function properly in an organism. Air moving too quickly because of too much space can result in diseases such as diarrhea, while Air being restricted by not enough space can result in constipation.

For each *doṣa*, Āyurveda lists twenty properties based on the relative strength of each *dosha* according to certain dualities. Of these dualities the most important are hot-cold, heavy-light, and moist-dry. The main qualities of the three *doṣas* — *pitta* (bile), *kapha* (phlegm), and *vata* (air) — are that compared to the other *doṣas pitta* is hotter, *vata* is drier, and *kapha* is heavier. From this we can understand that compared to *vata pitta* is not only hotter, but also moister, and compared to *kapha pitta* is lighter. In this way we can say that compared to the other *doṣas pitta* is hot, light, and moist; *vata* is dry, light, and cool; *kapha* is heavy, moist, and cool. According to Āyurveda, at the time of birth each living entity has a body composed of a proportion of these three *doṣas* called *janma prakṛti*. This *prakṛti* remains the same during one's entire life. One of the requirements for the body to be healthy is to maintain this balance of the *doṣas*. When a different proportion of *doṣas* arises in the body, this is called *vikriti*. For example, if at the time of birth a person's *doṣic* balance is V2P3K1 (*vata* 2, *pitta* 3, and *kapha* 1). We could say that at birth *vata* is twice as prominent in the body as *kapha*, and *pitta* is three times as prominent as *kapha*, while *pitta* is 1.5 times as prominent as *vata*. If at some point this doshic balance changes to V2P4K1, we can say that there is now an imbalance of *pitta* in the body.

In the material world, the seasons, the time of day, our activities, our consciousness, our diet, and our age have doshic qualities. The doshic qualities of these factors have an influence on the balance of the *doṣas* in our body and mind. For instance, in summer *pitta* predominates; in fall, *vata* predominates; in winter, *kapha* predominates, and in spring both *pitta* and *kapha* predominate. In the summer heat, the body tries to balance itself by removing excess heat from the body. Sweat, which carries the heat out of the body, is a combination of water and fire. Because there is less heat in the body, the fire of digestion also decreases. In the winter, when it is colder, fire is maintained within the body and the fire of digestion becomes stronger.

Because time changes everything in the material universe, the body constantly has to readjust to changing external and internal factors. The ability or inability of the body to readjust itself is determined by the strength of the immune system. During the day, as the sun rises and heats up our environment, the body must deal effectively with these changes to remain balanced. If the body cannot adjust itself, an imbalance of the *doṣas* will take place, and this imbalance is the beginning of a state of disease. Disease can be taken as a lack ("dis") of "ease."

Usually, one factor in our health we can readily control is our diet. Therefore, Āyurveda stresses being conscious of what we eat and how it effects our digestion. It is said in Āyurveda that food is what we can digest, medicine is what helps our digestion, and poison is what we cannot digest. One axiom or *sutra* in Āyurveda says, "Like increases like, and opposites balance each other." Every type of food has a certain unique balance of *doṣas* and properties which affect our bodies as well as our consciousness in different ways when eaten. Therefore, if we want to maintain a healthy balance of the *doṣas* in our body, we should choose the right kinds of food for our sustenance.

Knowing the science of what to eat, when to eat, and how to eat is a major factor in keeping good health. In our next article these subjects will be discussed further.

Āyurveda 102

In this article His Holiness Prahlādānanda Swami continues his series on Ayurveda, describing in more detail the science of what to eat, when to eat, and how to eat — this being a major factor in keeping us healthy.

There are two main physical boundaries that protect our bodies from external invaders — the skin and the digestive tract. Both of these systems stop potential marauders like germs or viruses getting into the bloodstream. In addition the gut stops undigested food from entering directly into our body's tissues — the food is processed and transformed before it becomes an integral part of the body. Otherwise, if there were a rupture in the gastrointestinal tract, and food entered into the body's cavities undigested, it would be treated as an alien invader and dealt with accordingly by the immune system. Thus, the immune system is another level of bodily defense that is controlled by material nature under the name of *ahaṅkāra*.[1] The body's most subtle defense system is the aura,

[1] "*ahaṅkāra*" in Sanskrit means "*aham*" — "I am, "*kāra*" — the doer." However, according to the *Bhagavad-gītā* (9.10), Lord Krishna is the actual doer, moving the material energy through his energy called *maya*. Lord Krishna says: "This material nature, which is one of My energies, is working under My direction, O son of Kunti, producing all moving and nonmoving beings. Under its rule this manifestation is created and annihilated again and again." Therefore, it is Lord Krishna who is really in control of the material energy. Nevertheless, material nature creates bodies for individual living entities whose material personalities are controlled by *ahaṅkāra*.

Though a living entity's body may comprise trillions of cells, in a healthy body they cooperate with one another under the command of this agency of the external energy. Again in the *Bhagavad-gītā* the Lord mentions that the living soul who is a particle of His spiritual energy is different from the material body. Our identification with the material body is called *ahamkara*.

So *ahamkara* is not unreal, but is the commander of the material body and maintains the sense of identity of its innumerable cells so that they work cooperatively. However, the soul's sense of being the commander of these cells is what is actually unreal, for the soul can simply desire, — it is the Supreme Lord who fulfill those his desires through the material energy.

Due to past activities, either in present or previous bodies, different desires arise within the mind of the soul conditioned by the material energy. When the soul has the intelligence to understand which desires are favorable for good health and which desires are not, he or she can decide to accept the favorable desires and not be influenced by those that are detrimental. That knowledge of what is favorable to good health and what is unfavorable is found in the Ayurvedic science.

which blocks unwelcomed negative vibrations from even entering into our consciousness. In a healthy body, disease does not take root because the digestion functions properly and the immune system and aura is strong.

As far as eating is concerned, it is important to understand that what we can digest and assimilate counts far more than what we eat. In Ayurveda, what we can digest is called "food," what we cannot digest is "poison," and what helps our digestion is "medicine." Digestion begins when food touches the tongue. This contact sends messages to the brain and stomach about what kind of food has been ingested, so the stomach prepares the proper gastric juices that contain the enzymes for digestion.

Disease usually begins when the digestive process becomes imbalanced and food is not properly digested. Instead of nutrients being produced from ingested food, āma, or toxins, are created. These toxins act as food for unwanted elements such as parasites, viruses, and germs, encouraging them to propagate and eventually overwhelm the bodily systems leading to various diseases. Our health depends upon acting with proper intelligence as well as following a suitable lifestyle and eating habits.

Generally, a living entity survives by eating other living entities. The main energy responsible for digestion of this food is the digestive fire, *agni*.

There are four different states of *agni*: 1) *sama*, 2) *vishagya*, 3) *tiksa*, and 4) *manda*.

1. *Sama agni* is when *agni* is balanced and digestion goes on in a regulated way with the essential materials of the food being assimilated by the body.
2. *Vishagya agni* is when the *agni* is variable. A person with such *agni* sometimes has constipation and sometimes diarrhea. *Vishagya agni* is usually associated with *vata* dosha.
3. *Tiksa agni* occurs when the fire of digestion is too high and thus the food and its essential parts are rapidly burned — thus even large meals are digested in a very short time. Although such a person may be continuously hungry, and eat large meals, little of the digested food is assimilated since most of it is incinerated. *Tiksa agni* is usually associated with *pitta* dosha.
4. *Manda agni* is slow digestion when food remains undigested and unassimilated. *Manda agni* is usually associated with *kapha* dosha.

Regulation of one's bodily necessities is an important method to achieve the balanced and healthy state of *sama-agni*. The importance of living a balanced lifestyle is confirmed by Lord Krishna in the *Bhagavad-gītä* (6.17): "He who is regulated in his habits of eating, sleeping, recreation and work can mitigate all material pains by practicing the yoga system."

Digested food is formed into seven different kinds of tissues that are the support of the body. These tissues are called the seven *dhätus*. They support the gross physical body and the subtle mind. The seven dhatus are: 1) *rasa* (plasma), 2) *rakta* (blood), 3) *maṁsa* (muscle), 4) *medas* (fat), 5) *asthi* (bones), 6) *majjä* (bone marrow), and 7) *śukra / ārtava* (the male and female reproductive system respectively). When the seven dhatus are strong and well formed then the digestive fires within the body remain in balance and the psychological processes that keep the body and mind healthy remain vigorous.

When food is eaten at regulated times and according to one's capacity, then it is converted into progressively more subtle and higher doshas culminating in *Ojas*. *Ojas* is the support for the energies of tejas and prana. Tejas controls all the subtle and gross fires within the body, and is responsible for digestion on the subtle and the gross physical platforms. *Präna*, on the other hand, supplies energy for movement and activity. If *ojas* is strong, the other subtle energies, tejas and prana, can work at full capacity within the body.

Ojas is formed as the essence of the reproductive system from sukra and arthava. If there is lack of digestion on the level of the dhatus (bodily tissues) then sukra and arthava will have some deficiencies.

In Issue 15 of *Hope This Meets You in Good Health*, my article "Ayurveda 101" gave details of the three doshas that a person's constitution is composed of. It also discussed the six tastes that comprise our everyday experiences physically, emotionally, and mentally.

There is a *sūtra*, a short saying, in Ayurveda that states, "like increases like and opposites balance each other." Our best doshic balance is the balance of doshas we had at the time of our birth. Good health throughout life depends on keeping as close as we can to that original balance of doshas. Our balance at the time of birth is called prakriti and any subsequent imbalance is called *vikṛiti*. If we have one dosha prominent in our constitution, there is a tendency to imbalance that *doṣa*. If there are two doshas equally prominent in our constitution there is a tendency to imbalance both doshas, or to minimize the lesser *doṣa.*

Keeping the doshas in balance is aided by a balanced lifestyle. Although in Ayurveda a balanced mental and emotional life is seen as having the greatest influence on the doshas, our physical activities are generally easier to control. Of the four important daily activities in life, namely eating, sleeping, mating, and defending, eating serves as the basic activity. Eating is the foundation for either balancing or unbalancing our *doṣas*.

Each *doṣic* energy keeps two of the basic elements in balance: *vata* — Air and Ether; *pitta* — Water and Fire; *kapha* — Water and Earth. The elements are general categories for the different material energies. For example, Air is the energy that moves all the other material elements. Fire is the energy that transforms all other energies from one state to another, such as transforming ice to water or water to steam. Water is the energy that is the "glue" that keeps different material elements together, like the water that holds together the flour when making dough for bread. Earth is the energy that produces solidity.

There are six tastes that are also composed of different material elements. As the following charts shows:

Taste	Elements
Sweet	Earth + Water
Sour	Earth + Fire
Salty	Water + Fire
Pungent	Air + Fire
Bitter	Air + Ether
Astringent	Air + Earth

The process of digestion produces the different doshas according to the tastes that we are eating. Our health depends on our regularly eliminating the *doṣas* and not creating an imbalance in them that would impede the process of digestion. The properties of the tastes depend on the elements of which they are comprised:

Sweet

In Sanskrit the word for sweet is *madhura* — this has a number of meanings such as agreeable, pleasant, melodious, and sweet. The main qualities of sweet are heavy, cooling, and oily. Sweet pacifies both *vata* and *pitta*, but increases *kapha*. The sweet taste is strongly present in all foods that contain sugar, as well as foods such as licorice. It is also present in the highest number of foods, and includes all foods that are considered carbohydrates such as grains, as well as foods such as milk. The amount of sweet taste found in any given food is relative. For example, a food such as rice may not appear sweet, but if something bitter is taken first and then some rice, the sweet quality of the rice will become more apparent.

The sweet taste is anabolic — it helps to build bodily tissues. It gives strength and stability to the body and enhances energy and vitality. It relieves hunger and thirst. Love is considered sweet, but too much sweet can cause stagnation and block the channels of the body. When the sweet taste is not properly digested it serves as food for pathogens such as viruses, bacteria, and parasites. Overindulgence in sweet taste can also thicken the blood and can lead to high cholesterol, high triglycerides, and narrowing of the arteries.

When in balance the sweet taste creates love and joy — the "sweet taste of success." When out of balance it can lead to greed, material complacency, and attachment.

Sour

The Earth element in the sour taste aides in building the body structure, the Fire element helps in digestion. In Sanskrit for sour is "amla," which means "acidic" and "that which easily ferments." Sour increases *pitta* and *kapha* and decreases *vata*. Its properties are liquid, light, heating, and oily. All fermented foods have the taste of sour as well as sour cream, yogurt, vinegar, citrus fruits such as lemon and grapefruit, green grapes, and unripe mango.

Sour, having the Fire element, sharpens the senses and aids digestion, it can also give a sense of refreshment and encourage the elimination of wastes. However, due to the presence of the Earth element it can also clog the channels of the body when used excessively. Especially in a person of *pitta* constitution it can cause acidity, heartburn, and diseases such as gastritis and ulcers. In cases such as diarrhea and dysentery it should be avoided.

Sour sharpens the consciousness and brings awareness and discrimination. Too much sour can increase envy and jealousy such as in the story of "the fox and the grapes" syndrome where the fox was jumping for some grapes, but when he could not reach them he declares "they are sour." Vasant Lad, a respected Ayurvedic physician, points out, "When a relationship ends, there is often a sour taste in the mouth, which is a sign of judgment and rejection."[2]

Salty

The Water element of the salty taste gives the quality of being laxative, the Fire element of being anti-spasmodic. Salty taste increases *pitta* and *kapha* and reduces *vata*. In moderation, the salty taste enhances the flavor of other foods. In excess it creates water retention. In very great excess, vomiting. It helps to reduce flatulence by removing gas from the colon. Salt is necessary to help keep the proper electrolyte balance in the body. In general salt softens and loosens the tissues. Salt is found in all kinds of forms from table to rock salt. It is also found in seaweed and tamari.

Too much salt may thicken the blood vessels and produce high blood pressure. It can also aggravate skin conditions. In general, use of mineral rock salt does not aggravate *pitta* as much as other kinds of salt such as sea salt.

In balance, the salty taste will tend to increase the zest for life and aid in increasing inquisitiveness. In excess the salty taste will create excessive "lust" such as the "Old Salt" sailor who comes back to port after a long sea journey looking to gratify his senses unrestrictedly.

Pungent

The pungent taste contains Fire and Air elements and is called *kaṭu* in Sanskrit. The Fire element heats the body and the Air element lightens and dries the body. The pungent taste increases *pitta* and *vata* and decreases *kapha*. Initially, it will decrease *vata* because of the warming effect of the Fire element on *vata*, however, longer use will tend to increase *vata* because of pungent's drying effect.

Spices such as chilies, ginger, cloves, and black pepper have the pungent taste. Foods such as garlic, onions, and radishes are also pungent.

The pungent taste will tend to improve appetite, help digestion,

[2] *Ayurvedic Text Book;* Vasant Lad

burn fat, and remove clots and stagnation from the body. In excess, however, it will cause burning sensations and thirst. In excess it will also dry out the reproductive elements in the body and cause sexual debility. Excessive use will also aggravate *vata* causing tremors, insomnia, and muscle pain.

Psychologically, pungent sharpens the mind and aids enthusiasm and determination. However, in excess it can increase anger and frustration as in a "pungent retort."

Bitter

The bitter taste, having the Air and Ether elements, is the lightest of all the tastes. Having these elements will tend to increase *vata*, but decrease *pitta* and *kapha*. Examples of the bitter taste are found in turmeric root, bitter melon, aloe vera, dandelion root, neem, and sandalwood. Although not a common taste in the modern western diet it is also found in coffee. Vasanta Lad says that, "Bitter taste improves all others tastes, because if you have a little bitter then any food will taste good."

Bitter is cleansing for the liver and reduces all kinds of toxins and heat in the body and kills germs. It can relieve high blood sugar. Because of its dry and light qualities it can help to kindle the fire of digestion.

However, in excess bitter can be very debilitating and drying to the body. It dries all sexual secretions thus promoting celibacy.

Bitter causes introversion and introspection. In excess it can create aversion and isolation within the mind. "The bitter taste of failure."

Astringent

Composed of Earth and Air, the astringent taste can be restricting and drying. It increases *vata* and decreases *pitta* and *kapha*. The astringent taste is found in food such as unripe bananas, beans, and chickpeas. Its binding properties are useful in cases of constipation, and aid in curing ulcers. But in excess it also dries the bodily fluids causing loss of sexual potency and lack of circulation.

Astringent tends to cause the mind to become introverted. However, in excess it can also scatter the mind and cause fear and anxiety.

As far as mixed tastes are concerned, if we cut an orange, which tastes both sweet and sour, in half and then after eating the first half eat something sweet like maple syrup or honey, the second half of the orange will taste more sour and less sweet than the first half. What has changed is that our ability to taste sweet has been satiated by the syrup or honey. Thus, while eating the second half of the orange, the sour taste in the orange becomes more prominent.

Effects of the Tastes on the *Doṣas*

	Effects		
Taste	Vata	Pitta	Kapha
Sweet	↓ (decreases)	↓	↑
Sour	↓	↑	↑
Salty	↓	↑	↑
Pungent	↑ (increases)	↑	↓
Bitter	↑	↓	↓
Astringent	↑	↓	↓

To summarize, health is achieved when: the doshas are balanced according to one's basic constitution (prakriti); the fire of digestion (*agni*) is balanced; and the soul coordinates his or her senses, mind, and intelligence to work in harmony with one another.

The effect of taste on the different cells will be explained in the next issue.

Āyurveda 103

Śrīpāda Prahlādānanda Swami continues his series on Ayurveda and describes the science of what to eat, when to eat, and how to eat — all major factors in remaining healthy.

As previously mentioned (see: *Hope This Meets You in Good Health*, Issue 16, 2010), food undergoes different kinds of digestive processes before it is assimilated and becomes a part of the *dhatus*, the bodily tissues or structures. Of course, it is important for these processes *what* we eat, but it is even more important what we can actually *digest*.

Our digestion begins in our mouth when the tongue tastes the *rasa* (taste, flavor) of the food and sends messages to the brain as to what kind of substance the digestive system should prepare for. When food enters the stomach, the kind of *vīryä* (energy) of the food is determined by whether the taste of the food adds to the fire of digestion or whether further energy is required from the body. Thus *vīryä* may be hot or cold. Hot *vīryä* adds to the digestive fire, while cold *vīryä* needs additional energy from the digestive system.

The food is further digested in the colon in a process called *vipāka*, or digestion conversion of food into a state for assimilation. Here the tastes are transformed, so that they have an effect on the *malas* (excreta), namely, stool, urine, and sweat. But the tastes can also be used as nutrition by both the cells and the *dhātus*. The following table shows how different tastes are transformed into the different *vipākas*:

Taste	Vipaka
Sweet	Sweet
Salty	Sweet
Sour	Sour
Pungent	Pungent
Bitter	Pungent
Astringent	Pungent

The sweet *vipaka* tends to enhance bodily nutrition and helps eliminating the *malas*, while the sour *vipaka* enhances digestion on the cellular level and increases the acidity of the bodily secretions (it may make the stools loose). Pungent *vipaka* increases the *vata dosha* and can cause constipation, for it impedes the flow of bodily excretions.

Prabhava

When different substances with the same *rasa*, *virya*, and *vipaka* have different properties this is called *prabhava*. In his book *Ayurvedic Textbook, Volume One*, Vasant Lad mentions that two teaspoons of ghee added to milk is a laxative, but ghee added in smaller quantities such as half a teaspoon is constipating. This is due to *prabhava*. He gives another example: Rock salt and sea salt both have a salty taste, heating *virya*, and sweet *vipaka*. However, sea salt increases *kapha dosha* more and is not good for hypertension, while rock salt will not cause hypertension.

Some suggestions for good eating habits

Good eating habits will also help us digest food more easily. Out of all the eating habits, not eating more than we can digest is essential. If you are an elephant, you should eat like an elephant; if you are an ant, you should eat like an ant. However, if an ant eats like and elephant or if an elephant eats like an ant, there will surely be difficulties. Furthermore, locally grown food that is ripe and in season is more digestible than canned food that is out of season or shipped in from some distant place.

Here are some other suggestions:

1. One should not eat again before the last meal has been completely digested. Undigested food in the digestive tract (stomach and intestines) can be ascertained the morning by examining the tongue, feces, and urine. If the tongue is thickly coated, it is a sign of accumulation of toxins in the digestive tract. Urine should be beer-colored. Turbid dark-colored foul-smelling urine and feces full of undigested food are other signs of toxins in the digestive tract.
2. When there are signs of indigestion, including lack of appetite and heaviness of the limbs, one should fast for a meal or a day and give

the digestive system a chance to recover and process the toxins. You could also sip a tea prepared from ginger and water. Actually, the real sign of your body being prepared to process new food is when you are genuinely hungry. Mental hunger for new stimulation is not the real hunger that one experiences when the body is healthy and the digestive fire is ready to consume new food. If you are not able to recognize what is hunger, fast for a day or two and you will be able to perceive what genuine hunger is.

3. In his book *Prakṛti" Your Ayurvedic Constitution*, Robert Svoboda suggests this: "Never eat when angry, depressed, bored, or otherwise emotionally unstable, or immediately after any physical exertion."
4. Prepare food as an offering to the Supreme Person. In the *Bhagavad-gita*, Lord Krishna states that one should prepare food for the satisfaction of the Supreme, otherwise one will be infected by lower states of consciousness and must subsequently suffer the reactions of karmic activities. As spiritual souls, we have come to the material world with the desire to dominate the material nature and each other. This bullying tendency is especially prominent in our desire to dominate other creatures by consuming them in the form of food. By preparing the food desired by the Supreme Lord, such as fruit, vegetables, and grains and offering them to Him for His satisfaction, gradually the desire to dominate material resources diminishes. Eating with this consciousness will bring us closer to the Supreme Person and more in harmony with His multifaceted energies.
5. One should eat in a clean, peaceful, pleasant environment, so that one will not be distracted in the mediation of eating.
6. Before eating take a shower or at least wash your face, hands, and feet.
7. Concentrate on eating and chewing the food. Food that is not chewed will not be digested and will result in *āma*, or toxic accumulation in the digestive tract, that will eventually enter into the vital organs and cause chronic diseases.
8. Talking should be avoided while eating, so that you can chew the food properly and concentrate on the food's taste. The taste of the food

contains *prana* and thus energizes the body and mind; it also provides clues as to the digestive juices needed for proper digestion. Too much talking also tends to mix excessive air with the food and thus increases the likelihood of poor digestion.

9. While eating, try to face east, the direction of the rising sun, the source of the Earth's heat and fire.
10. Eat with people you know and trust.
11. Eat with appreciation and gratitude.
12. Before you eat, it's best if your right nostril is functioning properly. This in turn will enhance the functioning the digestion system. To test which nostril functions better, hold your hand in front of your nostrils and breathe into the palm. The right nostril will also become prominent by hooking your left armpit around the arm of a chair or by in- and exhaling from the right nostril by covering the left one.
13. If you have a weak digestive fire, try chewing a slice or two of ginger with a sprinkle of lemon juice from a fresh lemon; it will help you kindle it.
14. When possible, eat with your hands. The hands sense the heat of the food and give subtle clues to the brain to aid in the digestive process.
15. Robert Svoboda suggests: "After eating, drinking a mixture of yogurt and water will help the digestive fire. Those with weak digestion can use non-fat yogurt and a 1:3 proportion of yogurt to water; those with stronger digestion may use normal yogurt in a proportion of up to 3:1 yogurt to water."
16. After the meal, you could take a short walk. Rinsing the eyes with water will cool down some of the fire in the eyes that comes from the eyes' connection with the digestive fire in the stomach. Defecation should not be encouraged, but passing urine after eating is a sign of good health. Avoid reading and doing any other activity, such as looking at a computer or television screen, within two hours of eating. These activities will strain the eyes. Also avoid exercise or any strenuous activity within an hour after eating.
17. If you are physically weak or have eaten too much, lie on your left side

for twenty minutes to increase the digestive fire — but do not sleep.

18. In some climates when there are exteremely high temperatures, such as India, it is sometimes better not to consume large quantities of food during the hottest time of the day, usually midday. In extreme heat, in order to balance the influence of the external heat from the environment, the body eliminates some internal heat through sweating. This usually weakens the body's fire of digestion
19. No matter how strong your digestive fire is, allow at least two hours between meals.

Diet and Consciousness
Their Effects on Spiritual and Material Health

Śrīla Prabhupāda gave many instructions to his students concerning their health. He often said that to cure our material disease and to get free from material contamination, chanting Hare Kṛṣṇa is the medicine and Kṛṣṇa prasadam is the diet. In another lecture, to indicate how much we should eat, he told us that "if you are elephant you eat hundred pounds, but if you are an ant you eat one grain. Don't eat hundred pounds imitating the elephant. . . But if you are actually elephant then you eat like elephant. But if you are ant, don't eat like elephant, then you'll be in trouble."[1]

Āyurveda, the Vedic science of health, gives further details concerning eating properly and also recommends purified consciousness to assist in the maintenance of health and the attainment of spiritual advancement. According to Āyurveda, our general health is influenced by three different types of constitutions derived from the Elements (solid, liquid, gaseous, luminous and ethereal), gunas (three material modes of nature--goodness, passion and ignorance) and the balance of energies, called doshas (Vata, Pitta, Kapha), which our body possesses. Vata regulates bodily movements, Pitta regulates transformations within the body, and Kapha regulates bodily stability. The predominance of bodily elements, gunas or doshas produces three different types of constitutions, which can be called physical, mental and doshic. Factors, such as the condition of the sperm and ovum, as well as the mentality of the parents at the time of conception, influence the elements of the physical body and the modes of nature (gunas) acquired by the soul at birth. The balance of the energies in the body is the doshic prakriti, and that is also influenced by the parent's balance of doshas at the time of conception and the mother's habits during gestation. For maintaining health, the balance of the three doshas is most important.

The Three Doshas: Keys to Health and Sickness

These three doshas control the life energies within the gross and subtle bodies, and according to the prominence of one or more of these energies, our constitution (or prakriti) is said to be a particular dosha, or a combination of them. For example, if Pitta is prominent in the father and mother at the time of conception, then a child will be born whose constitution is predominantly Pitta. If Pitta is prominent in the father and Vata in the mother, then a child with the mixed constitution of Pitta and Vata will be born. Vata controls all the life airs and thus governs movements and sensations of the nervous system, as well as anxiety. Pitta governs all transformations that take place within the body and is thus the principal energy governing the digestion of food and our ability to assimilate ideas. Kapha governs the structures within the body and thus the body's stability and mental satisfaction.

In the Sanskrit language, dosha means fault. Thus Vata, Pitta, and Kapha are called doshas because they have a tendency to become imbalanced. Within our bodies, their balance or imbalance mainly depends on our diet and emotions. Food and emotions both have six tastes, which are called rasas in Sanskrit. The six rasas are: sweet, sour, salty, pungent, astringent and bitter. When in balance or unbalance, these tastes produce different effects. For example, on the emotional platform, when these tastes are balanced, they produce satisfaction, discrimination, zest, excitement, introspection and the desire for improvement. However, when these emotions are excessive, they can produce complacency or greed, envy, hedonism, impatience or anger, insecurity, and grief. Each taste has its own properties which affect the doshas. For example, the bitter taste, being composed mainly of air and ether, is cooling and drying, being thus the taste that most balances Pitta, (which increases the heat of the body and its moisture).

It is valuable to understand our constitution; just as knowing what kind of vehicle we are driving lets us know what fuel to put into the tank and when to change the oil. For instance, if we are born with a Pitta prakriti, then throughout our lives we will have a tendency for Pitta to be imbalanced. Pitta helps to give discrimination, organizational ability, and good digestion; too much can produce rashes, ulcers, bleeding, anger, and irritation. By an appropriate life-style, a person with a Pitta prakriti can keep Pitta in balance and enhance the positive qualities of his nature. In this case, the sweet, astringent, and bitter tastes are emphasized since they are mainly cooling, drying and heavy (sweet), which balances Pitta's hot, moist, and light effects.

Balanced Diet of Food and Emotions

According to Ayurveda, a balanced diet is one in which there are all six tastes in a quantity appropriate for the person's constitution, physical and mental state, season of the year, and age. It is often found, however, that people overeat the sweet taste most; this is perhaps a compensation for a lack of sweetness in their emotional life. Śr□la Prabhupāda warned us not to eat too many sweets. He said in one lecture: "The ants are very much fond of being intoxicated. Therefore, they find out sweet, sugar. Sweet is intoxication. The liquor is made from sugar. Sugar is fermented with acid, sulfuric acid, and then it is distilled. That is liquor. Therefore too much sweet eating is prohibited."[2]

We can see the effect of our emotional cravings on our activities if we examine how the influence of the media and sign boards for the "good things" of life increases the salty emotions within a person, which increases their desire for sensory stimulation. However, if the person compares how he is enjoying with others who are enjoying, the sour taste may arise, producing envy. Then if the person's desires increase beyond his ability to satisfy them, the pungent taste arises, producing anger. The whole experience produces a bitter taste within the person, which leads him to crave the opposite taste, sweet, for balance.

These emotional desires can be satisfied by coming into contact with the sweetest and most complete person Sri Kṛṣṇa. Therefore, by increasing our Kṛṣṇa consciousness, our unnecessary material desires will also be satisfied. If we are emotionally stable, we are less likely to overeat (ati-āhāraḥ) and over-collect (prayāsaḥ), and what we do eat will balance and nourish our bodies.

It's Not What We Eat that Counts, It's What We Digest

What we eat is not as important as what we digest and assimilate into our bodies. Therefore, how much and what we eat should be determined by the condition of our digestive tracts. One quick way of determining the condition of the digestive tract is to look at the tongue. A good digestive tract is indicated by a clean tongue with a nice reddish color. Coating on the tongue indicates the presence of undigested food (ama or toxins) in the gastro-intestinal tract. A coating on the back of the tongue indicates ama in the large intestine, in the middle, in the small intestine, and a coating in the front of the tongue indicates ama in the stomach. Fire in a fireplace cannot burn properly in the presence of accumulated ashes. Therefore, the fireplace must first be cleaned. Similarly the digestive fire (agni) cannot burn brightly and digest our food if ama or undigested food is still present in our digestive tract. Fasting is a good way to clean the intestinal tract. This can be done with no food and water, or with water or juice. If one fasts, he shouldn't increase his sleeping, so a juice fast with energy to serve Śrī Kṛṣṇa is preferable to a complete fast while asleep. During a fast, the energy normally used for digestion is used to digest the toxins. Furthermore, the condition of the stool and urine indicates the state of the digestive fire. The urine should be clear and the stool should be of the consistency of an unripened banana. Cloudy urine and undigested food in the stool indicates a lack of the fire of digestion.

If the digestive fire is strong, one should feel hunger. If one does not know if he is hungry or not, he isn't. If one feels hunger, one should first see how much he can digest and eat half of that, leaving 1/4 of the stomach free for air and liquids. Every fire burns better in a clean place with sufficient air. Similarly the digestive fire burns better when the stomach is not filled to capacity. Two palmfuls of food should be sufficient, as the stomach is not much bigger than that. A burp is a warning that should be heeded.

Food should be prepared and served by persons who have a genuine desire to please the Supreme Lord and His devotees. The consciousness of the cooks and servers is also infused into the food and has an effect on the eater. It is said in the Ayurveda that the food, after eaten, is divided by the digestive system into one part, which forms the physical body, in another part, which is eliminated as waste, and a third part, which forms the mind. Thus the consciousness of the cook will influence the mind of the eater of the food. The consciousness of the cook will be influenced by the cleanliness and orderliness of the kitchen. Of course, if one eats prasadam while being absorbed in Kṛṣṇa consciousness, one will purify any undesirable quality the food may possess. The purifying quality of prasadam is that it is prepared, offered, served and eaten with love for Lord Kṛṣṇa. The more the quality of love is increased, the more everything becomes purified by complete absorption in Kṛṣṇa consciousness.

Tips for Devotional Meals

Our conditioned life in the material world is caused by our desire to dominate the material energy. This mentality can be diminished by devotional service, especially by taking prasadam in full Kṛṣṇa consciousness. The following are some suggestions to help us concentrate on eating with devotion:

1. We should not eat when not physically hungry, when emotionally upset, bored or after physical exertion.

2. Bathe before eating or at least wash the hands, face and feet. 3

3. Sit in a clean, peaceful place.

4. For those with weak digestion or who are enthusiastic about details, the digestion will function better if the right nostril is working stronger than the left. This can be easily accomplished by breathing through the right nostril for a few minutes.

5. When prasadam is ready, offer prayers to Lord Kṛṣṇa.

6. Following Śrīla Prabhupāda's example, for those whose digestion is weak, in order to increase the fire of digestion, one can take a little raw ginger with lemon juice and a pinch of rock salt.

7. Eating with the hands is recommended to send the information to the brain about the texture and temperature of the food.

8. Concentrate on eating. To avoid swallowing air, silence is recommended. If we talk, light conversation is best.

8. After eating, wash the hands, face and feet. Washing the eyes with water is soothing to the eyes, as heat caused by digestion can weaken the eyes.

9. Urinate, but do not encourage defecation.

10. One can then walk 100 steps, and if tired it is better to lie on the left side for twenty minutes. Avoid sleeping if possible, since this could slow down digestion.

11. Don't exercise for at least one hour after eating. It is best not to sleep or study for at least two hours.

12. It is best not to eat at night, as this may interfere with deep sleep and cause disturbing dreams. Especially avoid sour foods and sweets as well as melons and ice cream or cheese.

Endnotes:

1. Śrīla Prabhupāda, Bhagavad-gītā Lecture 6.16-24, February 17, 1969 Los Ángeles

2. Śrīla Prabhupāda, Bhagavad-gītā Lecture Aug 25, 1975 London

3. Concerning cleanliness, Śrīla Prabhupāda wrote to Rupanuga dasa in May 1972 that "All the presidents of our centers should see that all the members are strictly observing the brahminical standards, such as rising early, cleansing at least twice daily, reading profusely, attending arati, like that. You begin immediately this process. That is the main work of GBC. Sometimes we see that even they do not wash hands after eating. Even after drinking water we should wash hands. That is Śucī, Śucī means purest."

The Four Pillars of Treatment

In an ancient Ayurvedic text, *Charaka Saṁhitā*, four essential pillars of treatment are mentioned: the physician, the nurse, the medicine and the patient. The quality of these pillars greatly effects the outcome of the treatment. Another, even more important factor is the Supreme Lord. Prahlāda Maharājā says that the protection of a good physician (or of parents or a strong boat) is insufficient to assure one protection. The ultimate shelter is Lord Kṛṣṇa, and one protected by Him is actually protected. Lord Kṛṣṇa's supreme will also determines the presence or absence of these four pillars.

First, let's examine the basic qualifications of an effective physician. A physician should be learned in Ayurvedic texts (or whatever bona fide system of medicine he practises). He should also have practical experience. Because cure is effected by "*yukti*," or a combination of factors properly put together, theoretical knowledge alone is insufficient. To some degree, awareness of the various factors that cause disease and effect a cure is developed by the doctor's experience. Also, a physician should be pure in his habits and intentions. That means that he should be in the mode of goodness, know the scripture and possess the qualities of truthfulness, cleanliness, sense and mind control. Physicians in the modes of ignorance and passion have qualities born of laziness and material desires and will probably not have the sensitivity or intelligence to understand the required remedial measures to treat patients properly. Knowledge is born from the mode of goodness. Physicians greedy for material things, such as money or fame, will have agitated senses and minds and unclear intelligence. That will make it difficult for them to understand the psychological problems their patients may be experiencing.

Second, the nurse must understand the directions of the physician and carry them out accurately. A nurse must be dutiful and sympathetic to the patient as well as clean and pure in all aspects of duty and consciousness.

Third, the remedy should be pure and potent and correct according to time, place and circumstances. It must be administered at the right time and in proper doses. It should effect a cure in a variety of ways.

For instance, we should understand that anything which regulates and balances the digestive fire is medicine; anything that disturbs the digestive fire is poison; and anything that the digestive fire can digest and properly assimilate is food. However, one man's food is another man's poison. People suffering from a cold (a *kapha* imbalance) may benefit from hot spices, which increase the body's ability to digest or eliminate the mucus. Someone suffering from an ulcer (a *pitta* condition) will react to hot spices very differently. They will tend to aggravate his condition.

Fourth, the patient must be willing to do what is necessary to become cured or, at least, to improve his condition. He must try to understand and carefully follow the directions of the doctor and nurse and must not become overwhelmed by anxiety and fear. Negative emotions in themselves can cause complications. Sometimes patients are not very serious about actually being cured. Other obligations may take precedence over their physical or mental illness. *Charaka Saṁhitā* lists four types of people who will not become cured. Among them are someone who puts his career before his health and the religious fanatic. Such people cannot expect to have their problems remedied, and they are usually satisfied just to have the symptoms obscured.

Ayurveda is an ancient medical science that takes into account these four factors in the treatment of disease. Although at one time Ayurveda was a complete science what included detailed knowledge of surgery and psychiatry, major parts of the science have been lost in time because of such factors as invasions into India by different cultures. Therefore it is not always practical, especially outside India, to rely on Ayurveda to cure various types of physical or mental diseases.

There are, however, many types of medical treatment that are in harmony with Ayurveda and work on similar principles. Chinese medicine is similar in many aspects to Ayurveda; it deals with many of the same principles of physiology and treatment. For instance, *vata, pitta* and *kapha* correspond to yin, yang, and the blood. The concept of meridians and their effects on the body is similar in both systems of medicine. As one may have faith that Ayurveda will be more effective in dealing with chronic problems than allopathic medicine, similarly, one could also expect Chinese medicine and similar sciences to be effective in dealing with such problems.

Śrīla Prabhupāda seemed to prefer Ayurveda, but under some

circumstances he also took allopathic medicine, though not always according to the doctor's directions. Śrīla Prabhupāda wrote in one letter: "I may inform you that I am inclined toward Ayurvedic treatment. You can consult the Ayurvedic physician in Vrindavan who is a Gauḍīya Vaiṣṇava . . . Consult necessary physicians, and let me know what I am to do. In Mathurā there are undoubtedly many Ayurvedic physicians and many quacks also. Try to avoid the quacks." (letter to Hari Bhakta Nudāsa, June 1 1967)

Śrīla Prabhupāda sometimes mentioned that a bona fide physician must give both diet and medicine. Kṛṣṇa consciousness, which cures the disease of the repetition of old age, disease and death, also administers a diet. Śrīla Prabhupāda writes in the *Caitanya-caritāmṛta*: "A diseased person needs both proper medicine and a proper diet, and therefore the Kṛṣṇa consciousness movement supplies materially stricken people with the medicine of the chanting of the holy name, or the Hare Kṛṣṇa *maha-mantra*, and the diet of *prasāda*."

Everything that we eat affects us physically and mentally. How can a complete medical science not take into account what we eat? Indeed, a truly learned physician must know the effects of food on the patient as well as the influence of activities, the environment and consciousness.

Those factors must be analyzed especially as to how they affect the digestive fire of the patient. In Ayurveda, the gastro-intestinal tract is considered the origin of health and disease. Disease begins with an imbalance within the body, mental or physical, which cause an imbalance in the digestive fire. This leads to indigestion and then toxins, or āma, which in turn blocks the gross and subtle channels in the body. This blockage prevents nutrition from reaching the tissues and cells and stops waste products from being eliminated. Any medical science that does not takes these processes into account is an incomplete science and can do little good to correct the root cause of physical and mental disturbances.

Out of all the factors, the physician is said to be the primary factor in the treatment. In Ayurvedic science physicians ascertain how strong both the disease and the patient are and compare their strengths. They must also consider what the possible causes of the disease are, such as the imbalance of the patient's doshas, the wastes, the climate, and the patient's mental state. Of all those factors, the patient's mental state is the most important. Cure can be lasting only when the patient agrees to abide by the laws of nature.

A doctor must also know the prognosis of the disease. There are four prognoses of disease: those that are easily curable; those that are curable with difficulty; those that can be relieved; and those that are incurable. In Charaka Samhita it is mentioned that anyone who puts his career before his health is doomed to suffer repeated illness. Śrīla Prabhupāda generally took the practical and scriptural point of view toward health. He wrote to a disciple: "Therefore, whenever there is bodily trouble we may adopt the prescribed methods of medical science and depend upon Krishna for His Mercy. The best remedy, not only for Śyāmā Dasi but for everyone, is to consult some approved physician. But ultimately we have to depend on the Mercy of Krishna, so we should chant regularly, pray to Krishna to give us a chance to serve Him, and, if required, we may adopt the approved method of treatment. (Letter to Kīrtanānanda from Los Angeles, February 14 1969)

Reduction and Tonification

As an example to encourage his disciples to take care of their health, Śrīla Prabhupāda once cited in a letter[1] an incident in the life of Sanatana Goswāmī. While on his way to meet Lord Caitanya Mahāprabhu in Jagannatha Puri, Sanatana Goswāmī traveled through the Jharikhanda forest and had contacted a skin disease that oozed pus. When at Jagannatha Puri Lord Caitanya used to embrace Sanatana Goswāmī. Unfortunately the pus from the Goswāmī's body would ooze unto the body of the Lord. Thinking that he was offending Lord Caitanya, the Goswāmī wanted to commit suicide. Lord Caitanya, however, learning of the plan told the Goswāmī that he did not approve of it. He told him that his body already belonged to the Lord and should not be destroyed or used whimsically.

In Ayurveda there are many definitions of health, but the following aspects of health are important:

One should have the proper amount of energy in order to do one's work. Too much energy, especially moving in the wrong directions or in the wrong parts of the body can make for hyperexcitability, nervousness, tension and other disturbances. Too little energy can make for depression, inactivity, weakness and other types of physical and emotional lack physical and mental power. The right amount of energy used in the right way is characteristic of the mode of goodness, which is most conducive to spiritual progress.

[1] I am very much anxious to know how is your present condition of health. Please let me know if you are improving or if there is some disturbance still. We should always remember that our body is not for sense gratification; it is for Krishna's service only. And to render very good sound service to Krishna we should not neglect the upkeep of the body. We learn from an instance of Sanatana Goswāmī. He was sometimes very much sick on account of eczema, and he was therefore sometimes bleeding. But whenever Lord Caitanya met Sanatana Goswāmī, He used to embrace him in spite of Sanatana's request for Him not to touch him. Because of this. Sanatana Goswāmī later on decided to commit suicide so Lord Caitanya would not embrace him in his bloody condition. This plan was understood by Lord Caitanya, and He called Sanatana Goswāmī and said to him, "you have decided to end this body, but don't you know that this body belongs to Krishna? You have already dedicated your body to Krishna so how can you decide to end it?" So you must not neglect the upkeep of your body. This is the lesson we get from Lord Caitanya and Sanatana Goswāmī. Try to take care of your health in the best possible way.

(Letter to Rayarama, February 2, 1969)

The senses, mind, intelligence and the soul should be working in harmony. Our activities, our desires, our understanding and our spiritual aspirations should be working together for a common purpose.

The doshas, vata, pitta, and kapha[2] should be balanced according to the balance which was present at the time of birth (prakrti), and remedies to balance the tendency for imbalance enviably caused by the (vrkrti) which manifests due to the factors of age, climate, season and other unavoidable associations.

Elimination of the bodily wastes (malas such as sweat, urine and feces) should be regular and timely.

The spiritual aspirations of the devotee should dominate over other necessities and desires that arise due to material association. Cakra, the author of the Cakra Saṁhitā and one of the original authorities on Ayurveda, declares that a person can't be truly healthy unless he is also spiritually advanced. Unchecked and unregulated material desires will lead to prajñāparādha or violating the laws of material nature and the subsequent diseases and problems caused by the threefold miseries.[3]

The basic supporting structures of the body which govern the physiology of the body called the dhatus (lymph, blood, fat, flesh, bone, marrow and reproductive tissues) and their assessory tissues are properly formed and their wastes are timely eliminated.

If there are imbalances to these systems and energies in the bodies the result is that sufficient energy will not be supplied to the cells and the wastes of the cells will not be eliminated.

In the treatment of disease and the restoration of health a two-fold process is employed called reduction (*laṇghana*) and tonification (*bṛṁhaṇa*). *Laṇghana* means to make light and *bṛṁhaṇa* means to make heavy. Reduction therapy is to eliminate unwanted toxins (*āma*) from the digestive tract and tissues. This allows the proper flow of the energies in the body's metabolic pathways so that the nutrients, which are formed after the process of digestion, can nourish the tissues and the cells of

[2] Primordial energies:
Vata—governs all movements within the body, such as breathing.
Pitta—governs all transformations within the body such as digestion.
Kapha—governs all the structures within the body such as the organs.

[3] Adhyātmic—pertaining to the body and mind
Adhidaivic—pertaining to natural disturbances like earthquakes, tornadoes, hurricanes.
Adhibhautic—pertaining to other living entities like biting insects.

the body. Generally after reduction therapy is completed, tonification therapy is used to restore the body's strength and vitality .

Reduction is indicated at the acute stage of a disease and reduces the toxins and excessive doshas from the body so that the energies of the body may flow properly. Reduction can also be used to prevent deep seated toxins from disturbing the body in the future.

Rejuvenation therapies are usually applied after the toxins and excessive doshas are eliminated from the body. These therapies build up the dhatus and energy in the body so that not only the body may work efficiently but also that higher consciousness may be developed toward the mode of goodness if not spiritual awakening.

The doshas have specific sites from where they can be eliminated. For *vāta* the site of elimination is the large intestine, for *pitta*, the small intestine and for *kapha*, the stomach

Reduction therapy has two parts: palliation and purification. Palliation(*Śamana*) loosens the toxins from the tissues and reduces them. It also builds up the digestive fire and cleanses the gastrointestinal tract. Before purification is used, generally there is a period of palliation therapy, and then again after purification therapy is applied, another therapy is applied to balance the body's doshas and restore the digestive fire. Then tonification therapy is usually administrated. Palliation therapy has seven parts: Fasting from water, fasting from food, herbs and spices to loosen and burn the toxins, herbs and spices for digestion, sun bathing, exposure to wind, and exercise.

In purification therapy (*pañcakarma*), first it is necessary to get the toxins and doshas to flow to their respective sites of elimination in the gastrointestinal tract. This is done by oil massage (*snehana*) and sweating therapies (*svedana*). Eliminating them from the gastrointestinal tract is then done by the five karmas. To eliminate *kapha* the strong therapy, vomiting is required, to eliminate *vāta* a mild therapy of enemas is required and for *pitta* a moderate therapy is required, purgation.

It is unique feature of Ayurveda that it not only flushes out toxins from the organs, but it also has a system of guiding them to the sites where they can be removed from the body. In this way, they will not be deposited again in some other tissues in the body.

When the patient is strong and the disease is weak, purification therapy is indicated; when the disease is strong, but the patient is weak then palliation therapy is indicated. When the toxins and aggravated doshas are in the gastrointestinal tract, purification methods can be used; otherwise, first palliation therapy is used so that the toxins and aggravated doshas can be brought to their respective places for elimination.

Pañcakarma is an art and generally must be administed under professional care. Many factors have to be considered such as: the disease, strength and age of the patient, the season, the proper combination and order of therapies. This requires an expert doctor, nurse, and proper medical facilities. Done whimsically it may not produce the desired results or the patient may even be harmed.

One simple test to see the current toxicity of our body is to examine our tongue in the morning. If the tongue is pink and clear, the body is free from *āma* and toxins. If the tongue is coated, or a color other than pink, such as red or yellowish, the body's has toxins. Another test is to check the stools in the morning. If the stools sink, have a bad aroma or if they contain undigested food, this is a symptom that the digestion is not working optimally. The stools should be light brown and the consistency of a ripe banana. The urine should also be clear and the color of beer. Nausea or weakness of the limbs is another sign of the presence of impurities in the body.

The root cause of toxins building up in the body is a weak, too strong or irregular fire of digestion. To bring the fire of digestion back into balance skipping a meal or two might help. This gives the fire of digestion a rest and also allows it to digest any accumulation of *āma* in the body. If the problem is more severe a juice fast for three days might be beneficial. A fast on fruit juice or lemon and water is recommended. If this is too difficult fruit can be eaten, but not grains or vegetables. After three days boiled vegetables, vegetable juices or soups can be eaten. After six days of such fasting the regular diet can be resumed; however, white flour products, fried foods, cold milk and sweets should be avoided. If the problem is more chronic, visit a competent physician.

If we try to build on a shaky foundation, the building can not maintain for long. Therefore if we want to build our strength and vitality to perform devotional service to the Lord it should be based on a internally and externally clear and well functioning body.

Some Hints to Keep Healthy

One devotee recently sent me the following letter:

"Mahārajā, for a long time I've been trying to figure out how to keep my body in reasonable shape while not spending a huge amount of time doing so. Should I do yoga? Aerobics? Tai Chi? Join the Vrindaban Racquet Ball club? etc... I don't think I'm alone. Probably many devotees are thinking in a similar way, but don't have the time or desire (after all it's a QII, important but not urgent thing) to research on my own what to do. With so many of us getting on in years, and so many senior devotees getting sick there is a need for pertinent information.

Are the Western theories right? Is yoga the only really good idea for devotees? If so, how does one learn it properly? "Light on Yoga" looks complicated and time consuming to me, and the author stresses the need for a guru. What about running? Walking? What about diet? Should we just "take *prasādam* and die"? Or else eat bland boiled vegetables instead????"

Here are some helpful hints for the devotees:

The first suggestion is to take shelter of the holy name of Lord Krsna and avoid the ten offenses because Lord Krsna can bestow all benedicions what to speak of good health to one who becomes Krsna consciousness. Faithfully doing service in Krsna consciousness, can improve our health.

It is recommended in *Charaka Saṁhitā* that to cleanse the mind of material toxins that lead to prajñāparādha, or willfully violating the laws of nature, we should chant the holy names of God. The root cause of disease is mental contamination, which produces wrong actions, which in turn lead to physical problems. Mental contaminations such as attachment to material sense gratification, fear of the future, and anger over our inability to control material nature can all be nullified by taking shelter of Lord Krsna through His holy name:

vīta-rāga-bhaya-krodhā
man-mayā mām upāśritāḥ
bahavo jñāna-tapasā
pūtā mad-bhāvam āgatāḥ

Being freed from attachment, fear and anger, being fully absorbed in Me and taking refuge in Me, many, many persons in the past became purified by knowledge of Me—and thus they all attained transcendental love for Me. (*Bhagavad-gītā* 4.10)

Śrila Prabhupāda gives the example of Kardama Muni, who, by his association with Lord Krsna in Krsna consciousness, maintained his health although undergoing austerities:

"Generally yogis look very skinny because of their not being comfortably situated, but Kardama Muni was not emaciated, for he had seen the Supreme Personality of Godhead face to face. He looked healthy because he had directly received the nectarean sound vibrations from the lotus lips of the Personality of Godhead. Similarly, one who hears the transcendental sound vibration of the holy name of the Lord, Hare Krsna, also improves in health. We have actually seen that many *brahmacārīs* and *gṛhasthas* connected with the International Society for Krishna Consciousness have improved in health, and a luster has come to their faces. It is essential that a *brahmacārī* engaged in spiritual advancement look very healthy and lustrous.' (*Śrimad-Bhāgavatam* 3.21.45–47 purport)

In February 1975 Śrīla Prabhupāda wrote to a Mr. King and told him: "We practice bhakti-yoga strictly and since bhakti includes all other results obtained from practicing other yogas, as it is declared in the *Bhagavad-gītā* to be the culmination of all yogas it becomes unnecessary for us to apply any other techniques besides simply chanting and hearing about the Supreme Personality of Godhead, Krishna who is called Yogesvara or the master of all yoga. Of course, it is certain that if one sits with straight spine it may be of some help in his ability to concentrate, but it cannot be considered as essential by any means. That thing which is really essential in bhakti is to develop one's eternal dormant love for Krishna."

Effective medical treatment requires both medicine and proper diet. Śrila Prabhupāda often compared the chanting of the holy name to the proper medicine as stated in the Tenth Canto of *Śrimad-Bhāgavatam*. *Prasādam*, he declared is the transcendental diet to cure the disease of *bhava-roga*, the repetition of birth and death. "Although modern philanthropic physicians open gigantic hospitals, there are no hospitals to cure the material disease of the spirit soul. The Krsna consciousness movement has taken up the mission of curing this disease, but people are not very appreciative because they do not know what this disease is.

"A diseased person needs both proper medicine and a proper diet, and therefore the Krsna consciousness movement supplies materially stricken people with the medicine of the chanting of the holy name, or the Hare Krsna *mahā-mantra*, and the diet of *prasāda*. There are many hospitals and medical clinics to cure bodily diseases, but there are no such hospitals to cure the material disease of the spirit soul. The centers of the Kṛṣṇa consciousness movement are the only established hospitals that can cure man of birth, death, old age and disease." (*Caitanya-caritāmṛta, Ādi-līlā* 10.51 purport)

Although dancing during *kīrtana* is an excellent exercise, on one morning walk Śrila Prabhupāda mentioned that different hatha-yoga exercises are also good for health. These, or any other type of exercises, can only benefit if they are done regularly and with proper guidance. Starting and stopping exercise programs whimsically can do more harm than good. Therefore, a devotee should develop faith that all the results of other auspicious activities can be obtained by the practice of Krsna consciousness. At the same time he should do what is necessary to maintain his body in a state of health so he can execute his duties in Krsna consciousness.

The second suggestion is to avoid the causes of ill health.

In the *Śrimad-Bhāgavatam*, Śrila Prabhupāda has summarized the main causes of disease in this age: over-indulgence in sense gratification and irregular habits. Lack of regulation is the main cause of disease in Kali-yuga.

"In Kali-yuga, the duration of life is shortened not so much because of insufficient food but because of irregular habits. By keeping regular habits and eating simple food, any man can maintain his health. Overeating, over sense gratification, over dependence on another's mercy, and artificial standards of living sap the very vitality of human energy. Therefore the duration of life is shortened." (*Śrimad-Bhāgavatam*, 1.1.10, Purport)

I would advise the devotees to avoid regularly eating especially difficult to digest foods like fried, refined and very sweet food. When the food which we eat is not digested it turns into toxins (*āma*), which clogs the system and becomes the harbinger of disease. When we are clogged up, then fasting from a meal or a day or two is generally a good remedy. After fasting it is better not to feast, but to eat properly, according to our capacity.

In 1969 Śrila Prabhupāda wrote to Gargamuni saying: "I do not know what you are eating, but the eating program should be nutritious and simple, not luxurious.

That means *capatis*, *dāl*, vegetables, some butter, some fruits and milk. This is necessary for keeping good health. But we should not indulge in sweetballs or *halavā* or like that daily. Too much first-class eating may stimulate our sex desires, especially sweet preparations. Anyway, eat Krishna prasādam, but be careful that we may not indulge in luxury. For Krishna we can offer the most beautiful preparations, but for us *prasādam* should be very simple."

We should see that we take our meals at the right time and they should be appropriate for our body, our age, and the season. Śrila Prabhupāda once showed the example when he was discussing managment with one of his senior managers. When *prasādam* was brought in Śrila Prabhupāda stopped talking and become absorbed in taking prasādam without any further comments.

Proper and timely sleep is also important as Lord Krsna states in the Bhagavad-gita that one who is a yogi does not eat too much or too little, sleep to much or sleep too little. As suggested in the *Bhagavad-gītā*, one who is temperate in his material habits can minimize material pains and easily practice yoga. (*Bhagavad-gītā* 6. 16–17)

Another suggestion is not to be too anxious about health. Over-treatment of disease can also produce disease. Medicine should be taken with caution as the wrong medicine or the wrong amount of it can also imbalance the body. We should also remember that, although we want to maintain the body in a reasonable condition to serve Lord Krsna, health is not the goal of Krsna consciousness, nor can one stay healthy forever, as sooner or later, one must die. During a conversation in 1974, a nuclear scientist asked Śrila Prabhupāda about healing. Śrila Prabhupāda replied:

"There is no healing in the material world. There is disease always. There is no question of healing. Their healing is temporary. I am suffering from some disease. You give me some medicine. Does it mean that there will be no more disease? You heal that temporary disease. Again another disease. So where is the healing? So this is to be thought, that... Healing, that is the problem. There is no healing. There is always disease, this disease or that disease. If you prefer this disease [to] heal, you are cured, and there will be no more disease, then you are profited. Another disease.

You heal this, another disease. You heal this, another disease."

We should, however, avoid creating unnecessary suffering for ourselves. In the Chakara Samhita it mentions that there are different classes of persons who never will be healed. One group of such persons are those who put their work before their health. Who can help us if we over endeavor (*prayāsa*) in our work without considering the effects on our health, or put ourselves in situations of stress and refuse to take the time to compensate by relaxing? Lord Caitanaya told Sanatana Goswami that his body did not belong to him and since it belonged to Lord Krsna, he, Sanatana Goswami was obliged to protect and maintain it nicely.

Some other suggestions:

- Observe Ekadasi as strictly as possible by reducing eating or by fasting.
- Increase chanting and hearing and absorb the mind in Kṛṣṇa consciousness.
- Keep the body moving (exercise regularly) at least 5 to 10 minutes a day.
- Keep the bowels moving (keep your colon clean).
- Keep the breath moving (always breathe slowly and deeply). Take 5 minutes every day breathing quietly, deeply, and slowly to regenerate your stores of Prana.
- Chew your food slowly, avoid talking at meals, and concentrate on eating.
- Don't eat more than your stomach can hold (1/3 food, 1/3 water, 1/3 empty for heavy food) or (1/4 air, 1/2 food, 1/4 liquid for light food).
- Celibacy.
- Don't sleep immediately after meals; wait at least two hours.
- Avoid evacuating after eating, but try to urinate.
- If you are sick, see a recognized doctor. Don't play doctor or neglect your health.

Routine, a Secret of Health

What is the most important secret of health? *Śrīla Prabhupāda* reveals it in his purport to Srimad Bhagavatam 1.1.10:

"In Kali-yuga, the duration of life is shortened not so much because of unsufficient food but because of irregular habits. By keeping regular habits and eating simple food, any man can maintain his health. Overeating, over-sense gratification, over dependence on another's mercy, and artificial standards of living sap the very vitality of human energy. Therefore the duration of life is shortened."

Ayurveda explains that one of the main causes of ill health is stress. Stress can result from natural changes like the fall in temperature from day to night. When the stresses of material life occur, an imbalance in the body's energies (doshas) may prevent the body from adjusting adequately. The result is disease. Regulating our lives, however, will minimize the effect of stress, and therefore it may be said that the more regulated one's life, the healthier one will be.

To aid the regulation of life, Ayurveda prescribes daily and seasonal redulations.

The briefest possible healthy scenario would include:

1. Preparing the night before
2. Arising before dawn
3. Urination and defecation, to empty the digestive tract so that it has space to take in new nourishment.
4. Washing the hands, feet, face, mouth, eyes, and nose (all the senses), so that with purified sense organs we may accurately perceive the sense objects. Bathing.
5. Contemplation of the Deity.
6. Light massage, exercise
7. Breakfast

Sleep

A healthly morning regimen begins the night before, with sound sleep. Proper sleep has many benefits, such as helping to balance the energies of the body. Sleep gives complete rest to all the senses and the mind. Just as food helps restore carbohydrates, minerals, and other elements lost through physical exertion, sleep helps restore mental balance and gives freshness and inspiration to the mind. Deep sleep is a natural form of meditation.

Sleep not only helps maintain bodily weight, but also aids in the formation of *viryä*, a subtle energy, which gives the body luster and provides determination as well as intelligence.

One's work determines how much sleep one needs. A manual laborer will usually need more sleep than an office worker. As a general rule, the need for sleep declines with age. According to the Bhagavad-gita:

"One who eats more than required will dream very much while sleeping, and he must consequently sleep more than is required. One should not sleep more than six hours daily. One who sleeps more than six hours out of twenty-four in certainly influenced by the mode of ignorance. A person in the mode of ignorance is lazy and prone to sleep a great deal. Such a person cannot perform yoga."

(Bhagavad-gita 6.16, purport)

Elsewhere *Śrīla Prabhupāda* explains that different persons may require different amounts of sleep, but in any case one should try to minimize it: "Similarly, sleeping also. Sleep, you require some rest, but don't sleep twenty-six hours. Not like that. Utmost six hours to eight hours; sufficient for any healthy man. Even the doctor says, if anyone sleeps more than eight hours, he is diseased. He must be weak. Healthy man sleeps at a stretch six hours. That is sufficient. That's all. And those who are *tapasvīs*, they should reduce sleeping also. Just like the Goswamis did. Only one and a half hour or utmost two hours."

(Śrīmad Bhägavatam 1.5.35, Vrndavana, August 16, 1974)

Too much sleep can cause mental imbalances or such physical problems as indigestion, excessive yawning and disjointed limbs. One who has a severe throat problem, one who has been bitten by a snake, or one who has taken poison should sleep at night only under the direction of a qualified physician.

Irregular sleeping times can also create problems, such as sinusitis, headaches, loss of appetite, and even fever. One should generally not sleep during the day, but taking a nap during long summer day is okay.

Insufficient sleep can produce such symptoms as physical pain, heaviness in the head, yawning, indigestion, and drowsiness may cause insanity. According to Vagbhata, an authority on Ayurveda, "One who is celibate, who is not sensuous, and who is self-satisfied will get natural sleep at the proper time."

Insomniacs may try the following remedies:

1. Regular habits of eating, sleeping, work, and recreation can help overcome insomnia. Go to sleep at the same time each night, and wake up at the same time each morning.
2. Massaging the back of the head and neck and the soles of the feet with sesame oil (summer) or mustard oil (winter) can help induce sleep.
3. Take a warm bath.
4. Drink a cup of hot milk with 1/2 tsp of ghee.
5. Place one or two drops of oil in each ear.
6. Meditating on the Supreme Lord and His pastimes can induce peaceful sleep.
7. Physical labor helps induce sleep.

Physical exercise reduces mental strains, stresses, and anxieties, which may cause sleeplessness. When the brain is calm, sleep comes automatically.

Arising

Rising before sunrise has many benefits, one of which is that the body can more easily synchronize itself to the sun's rhythm. At the end of the night *vata* predominates, and its quality of lightness interferes with sound sleep. Since *vata* is also involved with elimination, it is best eliminate the wastes from the body before dawn.

Emptying the Digestive Tract

In a fireplace, a fire will burn best if you clean out the ashes first.Similarly, you will digest your food better if you can eliminate bodily wastes before eating.

Washing and Bathing

The skin is an important organ of elimination. Others, such as the kidneys and intestines, are less burdened and thus can more easily eliminate bodily wastes if the skin is eliminating normally. Regular bathing and washing greatly aids this process.

Meditation on the Deity.

As the body has to be purified, so does the mind. According to the Charaka Samhita, a standard Ayurvedic text, chanting the holy names of the Lord is the best way to purify the mind.

Light massage and exercise

The body has different channels, called srotas. When clear and open, these channels efficiently distribute nutrients to each cell in the body and draw off waste products. Exercise and massage help to open and cleanse these channels. When properly done, exercise also helps increase the intake of prana, or life force, within the body and mind. Thus exercise enlivens the senses, improves digestion, and produces a general sense of well-being.

Breakfast

Now that the body has been cleansed and the fire of digestion awakened, one can take food to provide energy for the day's activities. One should eat light during the warmer months and heavier during winter. This simple routine will help prevent disease and keep our energy level high so that we can perform our devotional service enthusiastically, free of mental and physical impediments.

Sadhana and Health

In the ancient Āyurvedic textbook, *Charak Samhitā*, it mentions that there are two important fundamental principles to obtain good health. One is to chant the names of God and the other is to eat food with devotion that is offered to the Supreme Lord. Therefore, even those aspiring for physical and mental health must understand that the basis of all health is spiritual consciousness. This spiritual consciousness can be developed when one performs regulated *sādhana* which helps the practitioner to become absorbed in spiritual values and awareness.

We find in the *Śrīmad-Bhāgavatam* that Kardama Muni, although he was engaged in fasting for an extended period of time, was able to keep excellent health because of his advanced Krishna consciousness,

"Entering that most sacred spot with his daughter and going near the sage, the first monarch, Svayambhuva Manu, saw the sage sitting in his hermitage, having just propitiated the sacred fire by pouring oblations into it. His body shone most brilliantly; though he had engaged in austere penance for a long time, he was not emaciated, for the Lord had cast His affectionate sidelong glance upon him and he had also heard the nectar flowing from the moonlike words of the Lord.

"The sage was tall, his eyes were large, like the petals of a lotus, and he had matted locks on his head. He was clad in rags. Svayambhuva Manu approached and saw him to be somewhat soiled, like an unpolished gem."

PURPORT
by His Divine Grace A.C. Bhaktivedanta Swami Prabhupāda

"Here are some descriptions of a *brahmacārī-yogī*. In the morning, the first duty of a *brahmacārī* seeking spiritual elevation is huta-hutasana, to offer sacrificial oblations to the Supreme Lord.

"Those engaged in *brahmacarya* cannot sleep until seven or nine o'clock in the morning. They must rise early in the morning, at least one and a half hours before the sun rises, and offer oblations, or in this age, they must chant the holy name of the Lord, Hare Krsna. As referred to by Lord Caitanya, *kalau nāsty eva nāsty eva nāsty eva gatir anyathā:* there is no other alternative, no other alternative, no other alternative, in this age, to chanting the holy name of the Lord. The *brahmacari* must rise early in the morning and, after placing himself, should chant the holy name of the Lord. From the very features of the sage, it appeared that he had undergone great austerities; that is the sign of one observing *brahmacarya*, the vow of celibacy. If one lives otherwise, it will be manifest in the lust visible in his face and body. The word *vidyotamānam* indicates that the *brahmacārī* feature showed in his body.

"That is the certificate that one has undergone great austerity in yoga. A drunkard or smoker or sex-monger can never be eligible to practice yoga. Generally yogis look very skinny because of their not being comfortably situated, but Kardama Muni was not emaciated, for he had seen the Supreme Personality of Godhead face to face. Here the word *snigdhāpāṅgāvalokanāt* means that he was fortunate enough to see the Supreme Lord face to face. He looked healthy because he had directly received the nectarean sound vibrations from the lotus lips of the Personality of Godhead. Similarly, one who hears the transcendental sound vibration of the holy name of the Lord, Hare Krsna, also improves in health. We have actually seen that many *brahmacārīs* and *gṛhasthas* connected with the International Society for Krishna Consciousness have improved in health, and a luster has come to their faces" (*Śrīmad-Bhāgavatam*, 3.21.45–47 verse and purport)

From the Āyurvedic point of view, the essence of the body's immune system is called *Ojas*. *Ojas* is perceivable in a healthy body as the body's glow. It is depicted in as a "halo" in some religious traditions. Our immune system supports the body's ability to maintain its necessary physiological functions and adapt to the stresses of an ever changing world and environment. *Ojas* is created from the essence of the reproductive system, which is formed by proper digestion of food by the other dhatus or physiological systems. *Ojas* maintains the subtle energies within the body such as tejas and prana.

These energies support the vital functions of the body. *Ojas* is dissipated from the body by mental anxiety and discharge of the body's reproductive fluids. The dissipation of *Ojas* from the body results amongst other things, in a lack of concentration, poor digestion, and poor immune response. The food that we eat generally takes about 45 days to transform from plasma to blood to other bodily forms to finally *Ojas*. However, there is one food, milk, that if properly digested within a day is transformed into *Ojas*.

There is another way that *Ojas* can be replenished, that is by meditation. The best meditation is on the names, forms, qualities, associates, and pastimes of the Supreme Lord. By proper sadhana one can fix the mind with devotion on Lord Sri Krishna and come under the internal potency of the Lord. A side benefit of such concentration on the Supreme is the formation of the energy of *Ojas* which if maintained by a regulated life assures proper health.

On the other hand, if one is not inclined to perform regulated sadhana in Krishna consciousness, it will be extremely difficult to avoid the influence of worldly association. Such worldly association tends to draw out and bring to the surface of our consciousness our dominant memories and desires from our previous activities, both in this life and in previous lives. Without the higher taste of Krishna consciousness it is likely that we will become attached to ideas of material enjoyment or the anxieties of material suffering. Such attachment to material ideas and desires leads us to material activities and the loss of spiritual discrimination. These in turn lead to irregular habits that decrease our health.

Śrīla Prabhupāda writes in the *Śrīmad-Bhāgavatam*:

"In Kali-yuga, the duration of life is shortened not so much because of insufficient food but because of irregular habits. By keeping regular habits and eating simple food, any man can maintain his health. Overeating, over-sense gratification, overdependence on another's mercy, and artificial standards of living, sap the very vitality of human energy. Therefore the duration of life is shortened." (*Śrīmad-Bhāgavatam* 1.1.10)

The conclusion is that the more we engage in regulated spiritual activities in Krishna consciousness, the more we become purified of the tendency to want to control and enjoy material nature.

Such purification helps us come to the spiritual level of consciousness where everything necessary for our devotional service is provided for us by the Supreme Lord, including material health.

Rules for Enlightenment and Happiness Yama and Niyama

It is estimated that as many as thirty million Americans regularly practice the physical and breathing exercises of *haṭha-yoga*. However, these exercises constitute only part of genuine yoga practice. They are two parts of an eightfold process called *aṣṭāṅga-yoga*. *Asta* means "eight," *aṅga* means "limbs," and *yoga* means "to link oneself with the Supreme." The foundation of *aṣṭāṅga-yoga* comprises the first two limbs, called *yama* and *niyama*, or social and personal duties. *Āsana* (physical postures) and *prāṇāyāma* (breathing exercises) are the third and fourth steps of the eightfold process. The remaining steps are *pratyāhāra* (detachment), *dhāraṇā* (contemplation), *dhyāna* (concentration), and *samādhi* (steady concentration).

Other processes of yoga—such as *bhakti-yoga*, the yoga of devotion—have rules and regulations similar to those of *aṣṭāṅga-yoga*. To reach the goals of yoga described by the authorities, one must follow a process of yoga systematically, just as to graduate from a school one must follow its curriculum. The foremost yoga authorities tell us that the ultimate goal of yoga is not to simply obtain health or personal powers but to realize ourselves as being different from matter, and ultimately to reestablish our dormant but eternal relationship with the Supreme Personality of Godhead.

All religious scriptures and yogic texts prescribe physical and mental disciplines for material and spiritual progress. Freedom from attachment and aversion arising out of the agitations of the mind and senses is possible only by following such discipline. In the ancient scripture from the *Vedas* called the *Bhagavad-gita*, our attachment to the three modes of material nature, called goodness, passion, and ignorance, is explained as the primary source of disturbance to our minds and bodies. It is the Supreme Lord who manifests and controls these modes through His potencies, and therefore one can overcome these modes only by a suitable process prescribed by the Lord. These modes influence us because of our desire to become the lord of the material creation, and also because of our frustration at our inability to become so. When our attachment to the lower modes and the propensities born from them diminishes, we gradually come to the mode of goodness, where the ignorance and sufferings of the lower modes diminish. When the pure spirit soul is entangled in illusion born out of the modes, it cannot perceive its original joyful nature. Any kind of yoga— whether *aṣṭāṅga* or *bhakti* (linking with the Supreme through acts of devotion)—is meant to help the soul become purified from the artificial covering of the modes of nature and revive its original consciousness.

Progressive yoga practice is a refinement of sense and mind control to develop pure intelligence. By a gradual development of spiritual intelligence, one can become situated on a platform beyond material conditioning. Thus we become free from the dictation of the material mind and senses. However, this state is only the preface to the actual platform of spiritual life, which begins when one awakens one's consciousness of the Supreme Personality of Godhead. After understanding oneself as Lord Krishna's eternal servant, one begins one's natural life of loving service in relationship with Him and His ever-liberated servants.

Generally there are two paths to reach perfection in yoga. The path of devotional service is the direct path while the indirect path involves renouncing the fruits of one's work, cultivating spiritual knowledge, practicing mediation on the Supreme Lord in the heart and then awakening devotion to the Lord. The indirect process is not recommended in this age called Kali because people are generally short-lived, irregular in their habits and without much physical or mental strength. Currently it may be possible for some exceptional men to reach perfection by the indirect process, but for people in general, it must be considered impossible. Those who are imitating the yoga system summarized by Lord Kṛṣṇa in the Bhagavad-gita, if they are not aware of the desired goal and the actual process of achieving it, will certainly waste their time.

The sage Patanjali, considered the father of *aṣṭāṅga-yoga,* explains the path in his book *Yoga Sutras*. These eight steps of the development of consciousness, known as *yama, niyama, āsana, prāṇāyāma, pratyāhāra, dhāraṇā, dhyāna,* and *samādhi* , are universal in that they manifest in some form in every activity. Suppose, for instance, someone is playing soccer (or, as it's known in most countries, football). *Yama* and *niyama* in regard to this sport could refer to what should be done and what should not be done. For instance, one should kick the ball, but not the referee. *Äsana* is the position the body should take in this activity, namely to strike the ball with the feet or head. Obviously, standing on one's head during this sport would not be advantageous. Next is *prāṇāyāma*, which generates energy, without which no one could play the game. *Pratyāhāra* refers to not becoming distracted by sensory stimulation. If during the game the fans are cheering a player running with the ball, he should not become distracted, stop, and put both his hands up to the crowd to acknowledge their appreciation. *Dhāraṇā* refers to contemplation. In soccer, knowing the positions of the ball, the other players, and the goal, along with other factors, is vital. *Dhyāna* means that one has to concentrate, in this case on kicking the ball toward the goal and avoiding opposing players. When a soccer player or his teammate kicks the ball through the goal, the whole team achieves (temporary) *samādhi*.

When we examine *yama* and *niyama* more closely, we find that Patanjali has divided them each into five categories:

Yama— social discipline
Ahimsa—nonviolence
Satya—truthfulness
Asteya—nonstealing
Brahmacarya—celibacy
Aparigraha—nonpossessiveness

Niyama— personal discipline
Śauca—cleanliness
Santoṣa—contentment
Tapas—austerity
Svādhyāya—study
Īśvara-praṇidhāna—surrender to God

The practice of controlling the senses and the mind by a process of discipline is also explained in the *Srimad Bhagavatam*:

tapasā brahmacaryeṇa
Śamena ca damena ca

tyāgena satya-Śaucābhyāṁ
yamena niyamena vā
deha-vāg-buddhijaṁ dhīrā
dharmajñāḥ Śraddhayānvitāḥ
kṣipanty aghaṁ mahad api
veṇu-gulmam ivānalaḥ

"To concentrate the mind, one must observe a life of celibacy and not fall down. One must undergo the austerity of voluntarily giving up sense enjoyment. One must then control the mind and senses, give charity, be truthful, clean and nonviolent, follow the regulative principles and regularly chant the holy name of the Lord. Thus a sober and faithful person who knows the religious principles is temporarily purified of all sins performed with his body, words and mind. These sins are like the dried leaves of creepers beneath a bamboo tree, which may be burned by fire although their roots remain to grow again at the first opportunity."(*Śrīmad-Bhāgavatam* B 6.1.13–14)

The Vaisnava restrictions of no illicit sex, meat-eating, gambling, or intoxication help develop positive qualities in the mode of goodness, such as cleanliness, mercy, truthfulness, and austerity, while following the spiritual practices such as regularly chanting the holy names of God help bring one to the transcendental level of awareness.

As *Śrīla Prabhupāda* explains in *the Nectar of Instruction*, text: 3

"As already explained, one should not be idle but should be very enthusiastic about executing the regulative principles—*tat-tat-karma-pravartana*. Neglect of the regulative principles will destroy devotional service. In this Krsna consciousness movement there are four basic regulative principles, forbidding illicit sex, meat-eating, gambling, and intoxication. A devotee must be very enthusiastic about following these principles. If he becomes slack in following any of them, his progress will certainly be checked. *Śrīla Rūpa Gosvāmī* therefore recommends, tat-*tat-karma-pravartanāt* : 'One must strictly follow the regulative principles of *vaidhi bhakti*.' In addition to these four prohibitions (*yama*), there are positive regulative principles (*niyama*), such as the daily chanting of sixteen rounds on *japa-mālā* beads. These regulative activities must be faithfully performed with enthusiasm. This is called *tat-tat-karma-pravartana*, or varied engagement in devotional service."

The good qualities developed by following the path of yoga, especially *bhakti-yoga* in Krishna consciousness, are further explained in the *Bhagavad-gita* (18.42) as:

Śamo damas tapaḥ Śaucaṁ
kṣāntir ārjavam eva ca
jñānaṁ vijñānam āstikyaṁ
brahma-karma svabhāva-jam

"Peacefulness, self-control, austerity, purity, tolerance, honesty, knowledge, wisdom and religiousness—these are the natural qualities by which the *brahmanas* work." (Bg 18.42)

The development of these qualities, although not the complete perfection of life, helps one come to the platform from which one becomes aware of the spiritual platform of experience and how to make spiritual progress in one's life.

We work first with our mind and intelligence then with our senses. If the mind and intelligence are engaged in material desires for sense gratification, our show of yogic practice will not bear any results. Temporarily or externally we may follow some discipline, but ultimately the thoughts of sense gratification will impel us to fulfill the demands of the mind and senses. It is therefore a misconception to think that performing *asanas* to reduce fat or for health is somehow a method of spiritual realization. The practice of physical exercises without proper discipline will not help one progress on any path of spiritual perfection. As Lord Krishna says in the *Bhagavad-gita* (3.6):

karmendriyāṇi saṁyamya
ya āste manasā smaran
indriyārthān vimūḍhātmā
mithyācāraḥ sa ucyate

"One who restrains the senses of action but whose mind dwells on sense objects certainly deludes himself and is called a pretender."

One may apparently achieve a certain degree of physical health by a physical process alone, but even this health will probably not be very long-lasting, just as a pot with a crack will not hold water for very long. Of all the principles, the principle of control of the tongue and genitals is the most fundamental. Unless one can regulate one's choice of food and sex life, there is no possibility of becoming free from material consciousness, without which spiritual progress cannot exist. Freedom from sex desire is explained by *Śrīla Prabhupāda* in the *Bhagavad-gita*:

"'The vow of *brahmacarya* is meant to help one completely abstain from sex indulgence in work, words and mind-at all times, under all circumstances, and in all places.' No one can perform correct yoga practice through sex indulgence. *Brahmacarya* is taught, therefore, from childhood, when one has no knowledge of sex life. Children at the age of five are sent to the *guru-kula*, or the place of the spiritual master, and the master trains the young boys in the strict discipline of becoming *brahmacaris*. Without such practice, no one can make advancement in any yoga, whether it be *dhyana, jñāna*, or *bhakti*. One who, however, follows the rules and regulations of married life, having a sexual relationship only with his wife (and that also under regulation), is also called a *brahmacari*. Such a restrained householder *brahmacari* may be accepted in the *bhakti* school, but the *jnana* and *dhyana* schools do not even admit householder *brahmacaris*. They require complete abstinence without compromise. In the *bhakti* school, a householder *brahmacari* is allowed controlled sex life because the cult of *bhakti-yoga* is so powerful that one automatically loses sexual attraction, being engaged in the superior service of the Lord. In the *Bhagavad-gita* (2.59) it is said:

viṣayā vinivartante
nirāhārasya dehinaḥ
rasa-varjaṁ raso 'py asya
paraṁ dṛṣṭvā nivartate

Whereas others are forced to restrain themselves from sense gratification, a devotee of the Lord automatically refrains because of superior taste. Other than the devotee, no one has any information of that superior taste." (*Bhagavad-gita* 6.13–14, purport)

Our choice of food is influenced by our tongue's impulses to taste palatable food, and our conceptions of life are influenced by what we choose to listen to with our ears and to vibrate with our tongues. Lord Krishna therefore advises us to regulate the tongue's activities by engaging them in His service by eating food offered to Him and engaging in *Krishna-katha*, or topics about the Supreme Lord.

For one who is not directly engaged in the serve of the Supreme Lord, moderation of the activities of the senses is recommended:

"There is no possibility of one's becoming a yogi, O Arjuna, if one eats too much or eats too little, sleeps too much or does not sleep enough. He who is regulated in his habits of eating, sleeping, recreation, and work can mitigate all material pains by practicing the yoga system." (*Bhagavad-gita* 6.16–17)

To follow these rules and regulations, one must learn tolerance and detachment. This *Śrīla Prabhupāda* describes in his purport to *Srimad-Bhagavatam* 6.1.13–14:

"In text 14 the word *dhīrāḥ*, meaning 'those who are undisturbed under all circumstances,' is very significant. Krsna tells Arjuna in *Bhagavad-gita* (2.14):

mātrā-sparŚās tu kaunteya
Śītoṣṇa-sukha-duḥkha-dāḥ
āgamāpāyino 'nityās
tāṁs titikṣasva bhārata /

'O son of Kunti, the nonpermanent appearance of happiness and distress, and their disappearance in due course, are like the appearance and disappearance of winter and summer seasons. They arise from sense perception, O scion of Bharata, and one must learn to tolerate them without being disturbed.'"

However, ultimately the secret of success in any yogic practice is to obtain a higher taste. In the material world everyone is seeking happiness. Happiness is part of the nature of the eternal soul. However, when happiness is equated with the unrestricted gratification of the demands of the material senses and mind, one is sure to become entangled in the subsequent painful reactions. Sense gratification is also limited and temporary. One can not enjoy it perpetually but must renounce it after some time. However, when one achieves the spiritual platform of consciousness, the happiness is said to be *rasāmṛta-sindhu*; it is perpetual and is like an unlimited ocean.

Those of us who are not nearing perfection in the yoga process cannot expect that the practice of restriction (*yama* and *niyama*) will in the beginning always be pleasant. A person who has jaundice will not experience sugar candy as being sweet, but instead will think that it has a bitter taste. Nevertheless, one treatment for jaundice is the regular consumption of sugar candy. When the disease is terminated, the patient once again tastes sugar candy as sweet.

Lord Krishna says in the *Bhagavad-gita 18.37:*

"That which in the beginning may be just like poison but at the end is just like nectar and which awakens one to self-realization is said to be happiness in the mode of goodness."

Śīla Prabhupāda writes in his commentary:

"In the pursuit of self-realization, one has to follow many rules and regulations to control the mind and the senses and to concentrate the mind on the self. All these procedures are very difficult, bitter like poison, but if one is successful in following the regulations and comes to the transcendental position, he begins to drink real nectar, and he enjoys life."

Therefore, the main rule and regulation for spiritual advancement is to always engage the mind in hearing and chanting about the name, form, qualities, associates, and pastimes of the Supreme Lord and to always engage our senses in His devotional service, beginning with eating the remnants of food lovingly offered to Him.

Pranayama

by Prahladananda Swami and Krodhasamani Dasi

Modern societies are full of anxious people moving ever more quickly. We live in Kali-yuga, an age characterized by increasing stress and disturbance. But no matter how frantic their lives, people ultimately want peace and happiness. The Vedic literature says that irregularities in our lives contribute to many of our afflictions, and it offers remedies to relieve our distress and calm our disturbed minds. Like good doctors, the Vedic scriptures give remedies that fit the needs and propensities of the patients.

Of all recommended Vedic remedies, the jewel is *bhakti-yoga*, a yoga based on hearing and chanting transcendental topics and pure sounds, which spiritualizes our lives and makes us devoted to the service of the Supreme Personality of Godhead, Lord Krishna. But for those not inclined to such exclusive devotion, the opportunity to remove stress and regain vitality is given through *pranayama:* exercising control (*ayama*) of the life force (*prana*). *Pranayama* is the fourth of eight steps in the *astanga-yoga* system, which destroys ignorance and awakens spiritual consciousness. Although the eightfold yoga system is not recommended for self-realization in Kali-yuga, two parts of it, namely *asana* and *pranayama*, are helpful in keeping the body healthy and vibrant. The vitality produced by *asana* and *pranayama* can assist in other processes of self-realization, including *bhakti-yoga*.

In a previous age, Dhruva Maharaja, a five-year-old prince, realized the Supreme Lord by intense processes of sense and mind control. His practice included regular *pranayama*. In the cream of the *Vedas, Srimad-Bhagavatam*, Dhruva Maharaja is described as following the directions of his guru, Narada Muni. He practiced *astanga-yoga*, and after six months was able to stand on one leg and stop breathing. In this way, he fully concentrated his mind on the Supreme Lord within his heart

Controlling the mind and senses by yoga practice gradually ends our false identification with our gross and subtle material bodies. This world is a distraction for the spirit soul, who is bewildered by the Lord's illusory energy. We misidentify ourselves with our material body, mind, intelligence, and ego and struggle to maintain them, though they are only covering us, like shirts and coats.

Lord Krishna, the attractive object for the devotee engaged in *bhakti-yoga,* is also the center of attraction in *astanga-yoga.* King Dhṛtarāṣṭra is described in the *Srimad-Bhagavatam* as focusing his mind on the Supersoul, Lord Krishna in the heart, and obtaining liberation from material nature by practicing *astanga-yoga.* He took to the process late in his life, but with so much determination that he obtained freedom from the bodily conception of life and left his material body at will. *Śrīla Prabhupāda* writes (*Bhag.* 1.13.54):

"The preliminary activities of yoga are *asana, pranayama,...*etc. Maharaja Dhṛtarāṣṭra was able to attain success in those preliminary actions because he was seated in a sanctified place and was concentrating upon one objective, namely the Supreme Personality of Godhead (Hari). Thus all his senses were being engaged in the service of the Lord. This process directly helps the devotee to get freedom from the contaminations of material nature."

Formerly, people knew how to fix their minds on the Supreme by doing *asanas* and *pranayama.* In *The Nectar of Devotion, Śrīla Prabhupāda* tells of a *brahmana* in ancient times who after hearing about the glories of serving the Supreme Lord in meditation, began regularly taking a bath in the sacred river Godavari and then concentrating his mind by the process of *pranayama.* By mentally worshiping God (*manasā-pūjā*) he would perform elaborate service to his Deities, such as bathing, dressing, and feeding Them. Serving Lord Krishna directly and serving Him in the form of an authoritative mental image are both equally spiritual. Thus the *brahmana* reached the perfection of life and eventually was brought to the kingdom of God.

Now, in Ayurveda, *prana* is an essential component of *vata,* one of three major physiological forces in the body. The other two main forces are *pitta* and *kapha. Vata, pitta, kapha* manifest subtlely as *prana, tejas,* and *Ojas,* respectively. *Prana* can be compared to the electrical sparks in the carburetor of a car; *tejas* to the transformation, through combustion, of the fuel into energy; and *Ojas* to the fuel.

Prana, an energy different from oxygen or air, is found in abundance in a clean atmosphere, in pure water, and in fresh food. We experience *prana* immediately when we eat a fresh fruit. If we are hungry and chew a ripe apple, we quickly feel a surge of energy in the body and mind. Although the actual physical assimilation of the apple takes place down in the digestive tract, simply chewing it extracts *prana* and enlivens the body and mind.

Prana takes five major and five minor forms within the body. (See the box for a description of these different airs and their properties.)

The Five Major Vāyus

Prana, the upward-flowing air, is located principally between the head and the chest and throat. It governs inhalation, swallowing, sneezing, and spitting. This *prana* rules over the other airs within the body. Its movement is generally inward, as it brings external food, water, and air within the body.

Udāna, the upward-moving air, is centered within the chest and moves within the throat. This energy aids in memory, strength, and will, and in vocal and other types of expression. It is the air that governs exhalation, and being upward moving it helps us obtain higher states of awareness and consciousness.

Samāna, the air that equalizes, balances different aspects of the inner and outer material body. It is found principally within the small intestine, where it governs digestion and the assimilation of nutrients.

Vyāna, centered in the heart, is the all-pervading air. It expands outward and allows the arms and legs to function properly.

Apāna, the downward-flowing air, has its principal location in the colon, between the abdomen and the anus. It governs elimination of urine and stool, sex, and menstruation and childbirth in women. *Apāna vayu* also aids in the elimination of toxins within the body and the nourishment of the fetus in the womb.

The Five Minor Vāyus

Devadatta is located in the nostrils and the mouth and governs yawning and sneezing.

kṛkara is located in the throat, governs thirst and hunger, and helps in digestion.

Kurma is located in the eyelids, governs the opening and closing of the eyes, and winking and blinking.

Naga is located in the mouth. It is responsible for belching and hiccuping.

Dhananjaya pervades the entire body, causes swelling, and helps in the absorption of food.

For the health of the anatomical and physiological bodies, *prana* must circulate properly within the body. Imbalances of the vital airs quickly manifest as disease. *Prana* may move too quickly or too slowly or in the wrong direction, or there may be too little *prana* in the body. For instance, if *apana*, the downward moving air between the navel and anus, moves too slow or in the wrong direction, then we feel constipated. If it moves too fast, diarrhea may occur. *Śrīla Prabhupāda* writes (*Bhāg.* 3.28.11):

"According to Ayur-vedic medical science the three items *kapha, pitta* and *vayu* (phlegm, bile and air) maintain the physiological condition of the body. Modern medical science does not accept this physiological analysis as valid, but the ancient Ayur-vedic process of treatment is based upon these items. Ayur-vedic treatment concerns itself with the cause of these three elements, which are mentioned in many places in the *Bhāgavatam* as the basic conditions of the body. Here it is recommended that by practicing the breathing process of *pranayama* one can be released from contamination created by the principal physiological elements, by concentrating the mind one can become free from sinful activities, and by withdrawing the senses one can free himself from material association."

Asanas contribute to the realignment of the gross material body, but *pranayama* especially deals with the proper flow of energies within the physiological body, so that the subtle body is cleansed and rejuvenated. Different kinds of *pranayama* help maintain the normal movement of *prana* and increase it for vitality and concentration. *Prana* is held within the body by the power of *Ojas*, the end product of digestion, which manifests from *sukra* (the male reproductive fluid) or *arthava* (the female reproductive fluid). If for some reason, such as excessive sexual activity or disease, *Ojas* is diminished, it will be difficult to conserve *prana* and *tejas*. With inadequate *prana*, all the body's activities will be slower or more erratic. And inadequate *tejas* will diminish the gross and subtle digestive transformations of material elements. *Pranayama* will most be effective in combination with a suitable environment, life style, and diet.

According to Patanjali, the father of yoga, when you can sit in a stable, comfortable position and meditate, you have perfected *asana*. This position is especially important for *pranayama*, which is a subtle activity. However, for us who are not practiced in *asanas*, our introduction to *pranayama* can be on a chair that supports the back or on the floor with a blanket. What follows is a simple practice of *pranayama* that can help calm the mind and increase the flow of energy:

Ujjāyī Pranayama

Guidelines: Best done after *asanas* have prepared the body. Usually properly supervised *asana* practice takes two years. Practice in the early morning or evening, in a room with adequate ventilation, and the stomach and bowels empty.

Caution: Do not continue practicing *pranayama* if the lungs become tired or irritated; instead lie down and relax.

Sit on a chair or lie on a lift, and for 5 to 10 minutes simply "watch the breath." The breath will change. It will shift, because you are adding consciousness to your breathing. It is like waiting for a birth. Just as one waits for the birth of a child, similarly the yogis "wait for the birth of the breath." At this point the senses are drawn inward, toward the lotus feet of the Supreme Lord in the heart.

Prashant Iyengar, the son of B. K. S. Iyengar, said, "The breath is not our own. We should receive the breath like a gift from God. When one receives a gift, he receives it with humility and gratitude. The breath keeps the body and soul together, so it is a great gift from the Lord, and the exhalations always represent surrendering to the Lord within and to His will."

Take the breath from the pelvic rim, right above the top of the thighs, near the navel, and draw the breath upward from there. Take a long, soft, smooth inhalation, as the breath goes upward (as though you are filling a container with fluid). Softly draw the navel back slightly, toward the spine and upward. Make the side ribs long (as if you are making room for the breath to enter the diaphragm). When the breath has almost reached the top, lift the sternum bone upward like a plateau. Keep the dome shape of the diaphragm, and make a long, soft, smooth, peaceful exhalation. Take regular breaths in between. Take only three *ujjāyī* breaths, with regular breaths in between, as you do not want to disturb the very delicate nervous system. Notice how your breath is not really like a normal breath: It is thicker and has almost a watery quality to it. That is the *prana* that you are getting in touch with.

After these three *ujjāyī* breaths, lie down, then move to a classical *Śavāsana,* lying down with the legs, trunk, and head straight, and arms out to the sides of the trunk. There is no lift under the lungs. Simply take *Śavāsana,* let go, and surrender to the Lord within, starting with the release of the nerves. B. K. S. Iyengar's daughter, Geeta, says, "Release and soften the nerve fibers of the upper inner arms, and release and soften the nerve fibers of the upper inner legs." Then draw the senses inward, and surrender those senses to the Supreme Lord, the Personality of Godhead, Lord Krishna, situated within.

Śavāsana also teaches us, on the psychological level, how to let go, not only physically but mentally (holding on to grudges, or fears, or anything that prevents us from advancing in our own *sadhana,* or spiritual practice). This is an important pose, as it gives one energy. It teaches one how to draw the *prana* inward, and it allows the brain to rest, and teaches how to let go on the psychological level.

Celibacy

Ayurveda describes the process of digestion of food in its different stages. Digestion of food first takes place in the stomach, small, and large intestines. After the food is digested in the gastro-intestinal tract, the first product is called chyle (rasa) or lymph. As digestion proceeds further by different physiological and chemical processes, part of the chyle is converted into blood (rakta), blood to fat (mamsa), fat to muscle (medha), muscle to bone (asthi), bone to marrow (majja), and from marrow is produced vital fluids, sukra [male semen and other reproductive elements] or arthava [female reproductive elements]."

From semen is produced "*Ojas*", an essential, vital energy that supports other subtle energies such as "*agni*" subtle fire and "vayu" subtle air. *Ojas* also supports the immune system and it can sometimes be seen as the aura surrounding a person. *Ojas* is a container that holds *agni* and vayu and does not allow them to dissipate.

When there is an excessive loss of semen the subtle energy of *Ojas* is also reduced and therefore consequently other subtle causes of digestion also diminish in the body. This, in turn, can cause within the body all kinds of digestive and assimilative power to be reduced. As digestive power is necessary for physical and mental energy as well as the avoidance of toxins forming due to incomplete digestion, eventually the physical and mental faculties will be diminished which may lead to degenerative diseases.

According to Ayurveda, there is a link between the excessive loss of the vital fluids and mental disorders such as Alzheimer's Disease and dementia. If one dissipates his or her vital fluids as the root of the energies in the body, *Ojas*, *agni* and vayu are diminished so does the purity of the body and its energetic functioning. The cells in the body become swamped with impurities (*āma*) and the nourishment for the bodily cells and organs decreases. This can lead to any disorder including mental ones.

The subtle energy of *Ojas* can be lost in many ways, especially in old age when the bodily fluids tend to become drier. The physical act of sex greatly reduces the vital fluids within the body. However, even on the mental platform *Ojas* can diminish just by thinking about sex. Activities performed on both the gross platform or on the subtle platform have their effects. Losses such as in the case of semen are easily perceivable, whereas more subtle energy loss can usually at first be more easily felt than observed.

Keeping Your Eyes Bright

Even for a devotee it is common sense to take care of the body that Lord Krsna has provided us with for our devotional service. Although devotees may follow principles of cleanliness and regulation that naturally nourish their health, when it comes to their eyes what do they do for them? Usually, nothing. In the modern computer age perhaps we have to consider taking more care of them. So many devotees are using computers and straining their eyes.

In this material body eyes use a major part of the brain's resources. Almost 40 percent of the brain's physical capacity is used for seeing. Four out of twelve cranial nerves are dedicated to sight, two more of these nerves are used for assisting the sense of sight. As compared to this, for digestion and the working of the heart only one nerve is used.

CVS, computer vision syndrome, is a label that indicates straining the eyes due to working at a computer. In a recent study is was discovered that 90% of employees who work for three hours a day or more at computers suffer from some form of eye trouble.

What to do? Some suggestions:

Make sure the lighting where you are working is adequate. Too much contrast in intensity of light between the computer screen and the environment will strain the eyes.

Avoid screen glare.

Don't stare at your work when concentrating on it, keep your gaze gentle, and close your eyes now and then for a few moments to relax them.

Sit in a position where the neck and body are relaxed while looking at the screen of the computer. Other workspace ergonomics should be considered.

Consider taking breaks from staring at the computer screen. Lack of blinking due to staring will dry the eyes out and may cause irritation.

A good healthy diet and exercise are also important for good healthy eyes and vision.

Get enough sunlight when possible. Sunlight is the source of prana and energy for the eyes and the body. However, avoid staring directly into the sun.

Ayurveda recommends that after eating take some water and put in your mouth. Leave it there a sometime and then put the water into your eyes. The eyes are a *pitta* or fire organ and when digestion begins the heat in the body increase with possible delirious effects on the eyes. Putting water in the eyes, especially saliva in the eyes, cools them.

After eating for an hour, avoid intensely using your eyes.

Eye relaxation can be a major help. For this a technique called palming can be helpful.

To practice palming sit in a upright position keeping the back and neck straight and the head still. Rub your hands together briskly to generate heat.

Gently close your eyes and cup your palms gently over your eyes without pressing them.

Breath naturally, but fully and relax for a few minutes.

Feel how your eyes are becoming soothed, refreshed and relaxed.

Let your eyes become completely passive.

Opening your eyes let them gaze softly into the darkness.

Finally, slide your fingertips softly down along your forehead, your eyelids, your nose, your cheeks, your lips and your chin.

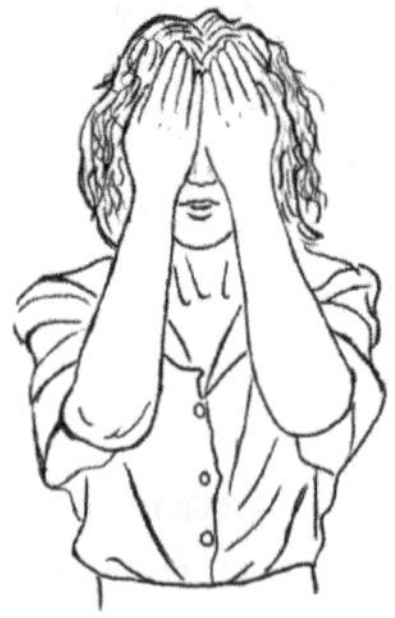

Exercise the eyes will help strengthen the eye muscles. Here is a simple one called "The Clock."

Imagine that you are gazing at the face of an old-fashioned clock with numbers and hands. See that the clock face fills the entire wall in front of you.

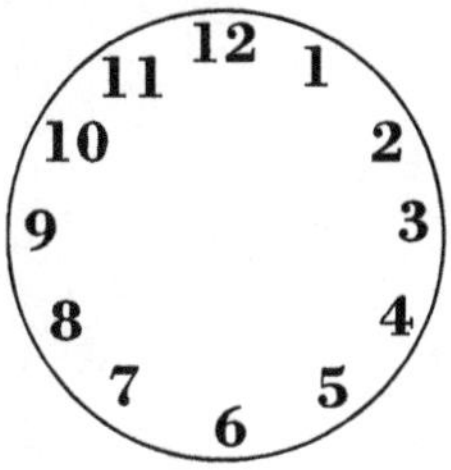

After each exercise, close your eyes for a few seconds and relax them.

Look up at 12 o'clock and then look down at 6 o'clock ten times up and down.
Look at 3 o'clock and then at 9 o'clock ten times back and forth.
Look at 11 o'clock and then at 5 o'clock ten times back and forth.
Look at 1 o'clock and then at 7 o'clock ten times back and forth.
Look at 10 o'clock and then at 4 o'clock ten times back and forth.
Look at 2 o'clock and then at 8 o'clock ten times back and forth.

Finally move your eyes all around on the outside of the clock ten times clockwise and then rest your eyes by palming and then ten times counter-clockwise ten times and then palm.

Tratak

Visualize the form of the Lord and His pastimes. This will strengthen the inner vision. Most of sight comes not from the brain, but from the internal workings of the mind. The eyes are receiving a billion impressions per second, but only a few are accepted by the mind.

Stare at a beautiful picture of Lord Krsna without blinking for 1–3 minutes. Your eyes will water, cleansing the eyes and tear ducts. Now close your eyes and visualize the picture in your mind. This will improve your eyesight, concentration and love for Lord Krsna.

For more detailed eye exercises there are books such as the Bates

Method and books by Sivananda Yoga that describe methods for not only relaxing and strengthening the muscles that aide in vision, but also for improving our visual acuity.

Try a few suggestions and see if you don't see the world in a new light.

The Alexander Technique and Krsna Consciousness

In 1978 I was traded from the American Radha-Damodar traveling party to the ISKCON Chicago temple to become the leader of the devotees who were distributing Śrīla Prabhupāda's books at O'Hare International Airport in Chicago. The Chicago airport provided unlimited engagement for book distributors, with more than 80,000 people passing through each day. Although my sales technique was still rough after nine years of book distribution, every day I was able to distribute sixty big books and collect the money to pay for them. The only problem was that I had to carry thirty or forty of those big books on my shoulder all day. Having only one book bag and little intelligence, I continued to carry the books only on my right shoulder for many months. Gradually the right side of my body became numb. Still, confident I was not my body, I kept going and felt that the service was more important than any bodily discomfort. After some time, however, I realized I would have to make some adjustments if I wanted to continue the service—and if I wanted to continue walking without crutches!

Thus I resumed a practice I had followed before joining ISKCON—*hatha-yoga*. When still a student at the University of Buffalo, in upstate New York, I had had a natural spiritual awakening, without the help of any drugs, and had realized that the purpose of life is to obtain higher consciousness. Within a month I had become a vegetarian—a fruitarian to be exact—and begun studying astrology and practicing *hatha-yoga*. One of my friends working as a model in an art school got me a job as a model doing *hatha-yoga* poses for a few hours a day. After becoming a devotee, however, I gave up such exercises as *maya* (illusion).

Now, in 1979, I took up *hatha-yoga* again, not to attain higher consciousness but to help me perform my devotional services, especially book distribution. And I have continued the practice ever since. My ability to do such services I owe to Lord Krsna's mercy and the help of many expert devotee yogis, especially two disciples of *Śrīla Prabhupāda*—Śyāmānanda Prabhu, who lives near Melbourne, and Krodhasamani-devi dasi, who has a yoga studio in Los Angeles, across from the LA temple.

Recently I visited a teacher of the Alexander Technique, Peter Grunwald, who lives in Auckland and who happens to be a cousin of His Holiness Tamal Krishna Goswami. Peter was recommended to me by His Holiness Devamrta Maharaja, who had benefited from the Alexander technique. I had visited Peter a couple of years earlier and found the experience pleasant, but at that time I could not fit the discipline of the Alexander Technique into my life. This time my experience was deeper.

Fredrick Matthias Alexander was born in Tasmania in 1869. He was a professional actor and gave dramatic recitations, which unfortunately resulted in a hoarse voice. After his voice completely failed him, he improved with rest and medication, but his voice failed again when he returned to the stage. Alexander was determined to find the underlying cause of his ailments. So, using mirrors, he examined his habits while reciting. One thing he discovered was that he was pulling his head back and down while reciting, which produced tension that resulted in various physical problems. After more careful observation, Alexander formulated many principles of balanced and healthy movement, which he taught widely, especially to actors, singers, musicians, dancers, and others involved in dramatic presentations. Both he and his students found that when the unwanted habits were corrected, many chronic ailments, often a result of poor breathing, automatically disappeared. The principles Alexander formulated are the basis of the school of the Alexander Technique.

In the Alexander Technique (AT), a teacher checks the student's response to a situation and guides him or her to first "inhibit" a response that gives an unsatisfactory result and then strive for a response that enables the student to perform the activity with minimum effort and tension and maximum of ease. AT teachers are trained to be very sensitive to changes in the body, whether the muscles are becoming tight or relaxed. They can also interpret the changes in the whole structure or through specific areas such as the voice or facial expression that result from such activities as walking, sitting, or speaking. The body functions properly when one performs activities with maximum efficiency, thus producing minimum mental and physical wear and tear and tension. In one sense, correct functioning simply involves the natural poise and movements unconditioned by acquired habits that are detrimental to proper usage of the body and mind. The one habit the Alexander Technique teaches is not to develop mindless habits, but to maintain mindfulness in all activities.

Peter Grunwald had practiced and taught the Alexander Technique for many years, and he had added his own insights, especially pertaining to the effect of eyesight and vision on poise and physiology. When I visited him in November, he began by asking me to visualize Lord Krsna and His pastimes, and by Peter's perception of the reactions of such meditations on me, both physically and visionally, he was able to evaluate the effects of different degrees of absorption in remembering Lord Krsna. Not surprisingly, the more I was able to visualize and feel the presence in a state of depth perception of Lord Krsna and His associates, the more coordination, ease of movement and poise Peter saw and perceived with his guiding hands. I was encouraged to understand more about the beneficial connection on many levels between Krsna consciousness and the practical ability to execute devotional service.

This experience was not an inspiration to try artificially to remember Lord Krsna, but an encouragement to perform devotional service in such a way that remembrance of Lord Krsna would come naturally in day-to-day activities. In the course Peter's instructions, I was reminded of *Śrīla Prabhupāda*, who from the first moment I saw him seemed to be a person with perfect poise. As a matter of fact, the first time I saw him he seemed to be floating down the corridor in the airport where he had just arrived!

Absorption in material sensory experience causes one to develop habits that prevent one from acting naturally or thinking rationally. Consider devotees who go out on book distribution for the first time. They are not sure what to say or how to respond to different people. This may create anxiety and tension that disturb their concentration (what Alexander called "end gaining"), and therefore when the approach people they are not relaxed and able to think quickly enough to capture people's interest and attention. By putting the situation in a Krsna conscious perspective, the inexperienced book distributor can become detached from the results and thus be less disturbed by what may or not happen when he approaches someone. This attitude will allow him or her to become more receptive to act as an instrument for the Supersoul within the heart, who supplies intelligence according to the qualifications, mood, and the sincerity of the devotees who are trying to serve Him.

Because many factors determine the results of any activity, a book may or may not be distributed, but the consciousness of being connected with Lord Krsna will certainly be there more easily, consistently, and profoundly. As a devotee becomes more confident and at ease with himself and others while engaged in such a service, he or she will certainly attract and interest many people to his or her message because they will see his or her inner and outer satisfaction. If we added to this a sincere feeling on the part of the devotee to serve and benefit others and a genuine appreciation for *Śrīla Prabhupāda*'s literatures, we have a winning combination for successful and steady book distribution and the development of Krsna consciousness.

The methodology F. M. Alexander developed is similar to Krsna consciousness in that he knowingly or unknowingly tried to get in touch with the pure intelligence coming from the Supersoul. His objective was to understand what was impeding his proper functioning in performing different activities (tensing his neck, for example). He was able to discover the poise that comes from giving up unnecessary tensions. By the grace of the Supersoul and the Alexander teacher, Peter Grunwald, I was able to reconfirm the grace and poise on all levels of existence that can come from the Supreme Lord when one serves and meditates on Him through the process of devotional service.

Peter Grunwald lives in Auckland, New Zealand with his wife and family. For futher reference regarding the Alexander Technque or finding a teacher, you can contact Peter at P.Grunwald@clear.net.nz.

Astrology and Ayurveda

Ayurveda and Vedic Astrology, Jyotisa, deal with the science of life. Indeed, Jyotisa means illumination through which we can understand our existence. Through the knowledge given in Ayurveda we can learn to live in harmony with the Supreme and His nature. Although we may misidentify ourselves with our material bodies or minds. We are actually spiritual souls within a material body. As a spiritual being we desire happiness and security. Ayurveda and Jyotish give the conditioned soul, whose consciousness has become influenced by material energy called the modes of material nature—goodness, passion and ignorance–information about how to live happily in this material world and at the same time progress towards different kinds of liberation. One kind of liberation is realization of our spiritual nature. However, the supreme liberation is in the awakening of our eternal body and identity and the reestablishment of our spiritual relationship with the all-attractive Supreme Person, who is called Lord Krishna in Sanskrit.

Among the different indicators in the science of jyotisa there are different planets that represent the different aspects of this world including their natures and interactions. These planets are the Sun, Moon, Jupiter, Saturn, Mars, Venus and Mercury. Rahu and Ketu also play significant roles in the soul's quest for spiritual or material perfection.

Generally, the conditioned souls imagine that some material arrangement can provide them with peace and happiness. One's identification is represented by the Sun in an astrological chart. When the identification is directed to the material body or mind it is called false ego. When the identification is directed as a servant of the Supreme it is called self-realization. The Sun in the horoscope also indicates how the soul will strive for peace and happiness by sacrifice and surrender in the material world. As the Sun is understood as the center of the universe that we live in, so in conditioned life the soul's false ego is the center of his existence. The conditioned soul's qualities and desires which are represented by other planets and their placements in the chart all revolve around the Sun situation. If the Sun is strong and well placed, sacrifice for higher causes comes naturally to such person. If the Sun is weak and ill-placed, one's personal fulfillment becomes the center of the person's efforts, even at the cost of the well-being of others .

Identifying oneself with the material world, the soul's consciousness further descents into material existence through the mind. The subtle material mind is represented in one's horoscope by the Moon. The mind's function is in the world of thinking, feeling, and willing. As with any planet, the effect of the Moon is in one's chart will be determined by its strength, placement, the houses and constellations it owns and other influences such as the planets that aspect it by their astrological glances. In the ever changing and unpredictable world, the conditioned mind naturally strives to have a stable, peaceful mind, which are the preliminary qualities necessary to find happiness. There are endless paths the soul follows in its attempts to find peace and happiness in the material world. Sometimes one may attempt to find peace and satisfaction through trying to satisfy one's desires, sometimes by tolerance and detachment, sometimes through sublimating one's desires and sometimes by transcending one desires and redirecting them to a higher state.

While the Sun in the astrological chart indicates our power and influence, the Moon in the chart represents where we feel most sensitive and vulnerable. The Moon rules the sign of Cancer so where Cancer fall in the astrological chart will indicate the areas of life where we feel most weakness and vulnerability. We try to compensate for these weaknesses by our strengths that are indicated by the Sun and the Sun's sign Leo. The Sun and its sign Leo establish how we can first establish peace in our lives and hearts through strengthening the sensitive area of life ruled by the Moon and then where and how we are willing to make sacrifices to fulfill our desires to obtain happiness.

The situation of the Moon and the sign it rules, Cancer, indicate where we must practice tolerance without invoking fear and overcompensation though our strengths as indicated by the Sun and Leo. The higher nature of the Sun manifest in directing our activities in the material world in a way that allows the soul's spiritual nature to manifest. The higher nature of the Moon allows for the tolerance and peace that keeps one on the spiritual path. When the soul's higher spiritual nature shines above the dualities of the material existence, the cultivation of higher spiritual wisdom and devotion proceeds without obstruction.

The Jupiter's placement and the signs that it rules in the chart indicate represents the soul's desire to expand into material existence in its quest for peace and happiness. Such expansion can be seen through visible creations such as children or material positions of authority or more subtly as one's qualities such as wisdom and optimism. On the higher plane Jupiter will give us wisdom to use our resources and abilities for spiritual cultivation. However, when Jupiter directs us towards our lower nature, he will inspire us to seek peace and happiness through material acquisitions, profit, adoration and distinction. When the soul's consciousness is covered by illusion, he is impelled by the lower modes of material nature to seek different arrangements though children and wealth to create a sense of protection and immortality. However, such material "soldiers" ultimately will prove inadequate security and defense against the inevitability of old age, disease, and death. Thus the soul will be again placed in another material body with another material situation in which he will again strive for happiness. However, no matter how intelligent he becomes and no matter how materially auspicious his situation, his ultimate goal of knowledge of how to obtain eternal happiness can not be fulfilled.

To accomplish whatever the soul's path to happiness in the material world effort, discipline and organization are required. Saturn represents the discipline and ability to create organization in one's life in order to fulfill one's objectives. The higher Saturn is the yogi in meditation controlling his lower desires while he does his duties to fulfill a higher purpose. For such a determined person it matters not if the duty is pleasant or unpleasant, but it must be done with patience and determination until the goal is reached. When influenced by the lower qualities of Saturn the soul attempts to control and manipulate the material energy to satisfy selfish and degraded desires.

In order to fulfill our duty we require the power, courage and determination manifested by the higher nature of Mars. The higher Mars is our courage to tolerate any adversity that stands in our way of discovering the truth and fulfilling our higher purposes in life. Influenced by the lower nature of Mars the soul becomes fearful and frustrated in his attempt to overcome the obstacles that he may confront to satisfy his goals.

Even if our path in life, our duties, and our determination are clear and strong, still to stay on our path we need devotion to experience beauty, harmony and a higher taste. Venus represents one's ability to see beauty and harmony through wisdom and appreciation. This higher taste comes from devotion to the Supreme and ability to see His creation and work in harmony with it. The soul influenced by the lower qualities of Venus seeks to gratify his senses with whatever the conditioned soul has available.

Now with our path of life clear, our duties systematically performed, our determination and courage set in place and our devotion steadily maintained, next the practical energy of Mercury comes into play to assimilate our qualities and efforts to manifest our desires in some concrete form. Mercury represents, our ability to discriminate, communicate, and assimilate. On the higher plane Mercury combines with our knowledge to manifest detached and renounced work allowing the qualities of the other planets to flow in one's life and thus create concrete manifestations. Influenced by the lower Mercury the soul will become distracted by by misdirected and uncontrolled curiosity in his attempt to experience the multifaceted creations and try to enjoy them though one's senses.

When Mercury is strengthened by clear goals, strong sense of duty, fearless determination, and devotional strength, then the aim of Jupiter towards higher consciousness leading to peace and awakening of one's real identity are fulfilled. When the intelligence of Mercury is defused into a dis-unified conception of life based on what will satisfy one's senses, the plans of Jupiter and the use of positive qualities of the other planets to find peace and self-realization are frustrated or forgotten.

So in summary we have different planets and their influences on the consciousness of the soul:

Sun ego (one's identity)

Moon Mind (desire for peace)

Jupiter (mission how to achieve peace and happiness)

Saturn (duties to be done to achieve mission)

Mars (determination, conviction, and courage to perform duties)

Venus (enthusiasm required to achieve goal)

Mercury (results that come from assimilation of the qualities of the planets to achieve one's goals)

When the soul misidentifies itself as a product of matter, peace and happiness is sought through sense gratification and material influence and power. In the Vedic culture there are four purposes of life: dharma, *artha*, *kama* and *moksa*. Dharma is one's duties according to one's psychophysical nature. *Artha* is one's attempt to obtain the material resources necessary to fulfill one's desires, *Kama*. *Moksa* is the freedom from material identification and ultimately the reestablishment of one's relationship with Lord Krishna.

In modern society artha and kama have become very prominent with hardly any if any idea of dharma and moksa. Generally, money and material influence and control is seen as the desirable outcome of endeavors. However, if one's activities do not help one understand and realize one's spiritual position then whatever the result may be, good or bad, one will not experience true peace and happiness. What will be produced, however, are the creation of more material desires and activities to fulfill them.

If one's spiritual identity is strong, although the other aspects of one's life may not be strongly supporting one's spiritual path, if one makes sincere endeavor the Supreme Lord will strengthen and purify one so that the spiritual realization will proceed with fewer impediments. However, if one is not spiritually strong enough, one may become distracted and not sufficiently be convinced and determined to rely upon the Supreme to help make up one's weaknesses.

One area of life that may cause impediments is that of disease. Disease can be taken as an indicator where we need more wisdom and balance in life.

In Ayurveda the main cause of disease is *prajnaparadha*. *Prajna* is wisdom and *aparadha* is an offense. This means not working in harmony with the material nature. When our desires are in harmony with the Supreme and His energies, then our plans, duties and disciplines produce acts of devotion that lead to spiritual activities and awakening. Thus satisfied with spiritual happiness the soul does not become addicted to happiness obtained through sensual experience and thus can refrain from excessive and unnecessary sensual gratifications. Being moderate in his habits, Lord Krishna says in the Bhagavad-Gita that such a *yogi* can mitigate the miseries arising from material contact.

Sanskrit Pronunciation Guide

Throughout the centuries, the Sanskrit language has been written in a variety of alphabets. The mode of writing most widely used throughout India, however, is called *devanagri*, which means, literally, the writing used in "the cities of the demigods." The *devanagri* alphabet consists of forty-eight characters: thirteen vowels and thirty-five consonants. Ancient Sanskrit grammarians arranged this alphabet according to practical linguistic principles, and this order has been accepted by all Western scholars. The system of transliteration used in this book conforms to a system that scholars have accepted to indicate the pronunciation of each Sanskrit sound.

The vowels are pronounced as follows:

Sr.no		Sr.no	
1.	a - as in but	7.	ṛ - as in rim
2.	ā - as in far but held twice as long as a	8.	ṝ - as in reed but held twice as long as ṛ
3.	i - as in pin	9.	ḹ - as in happily=
4.	ī - as in pique but held twice as long is i	10.	e - as in they
5.	u - as in push	11.	ai - as in aisle
6.	ū - as in rule but held twice as long as u	12.	o - as go
		13.	au – as how

The consonants are pronounced as follows:

Sr.no	**Gutterals** (pronounced from the throat)	Sr.no	**Palatals** (pronounced with the middle of the tongue against the palate)
14.	**k** - as in **k**ite	19.	**c** - as in **ch**air
15.	**kh** - as in Ec**kh**art	20.	**ch** - as in staun**ch-h**eart
16.	**g** - as in **g**ive	21.	**j** - as in **j**oy
17.	**gh** - as in di**g-h**ard	22.	**jh** - as in he**dgeh**og
18.	**ṇ** - as in si**ng**	23.	**ñ** - as in ca**ny**on

Sr.no	**Cerebrals** (pronounced with the tip of the tongue against the roof of the mouth)	Sr.no	**Dentals** (pronounced like the cerebrals but with the tongue against the teeth)
24.	**ṭ** - as in **t**ub	29.	**t** – **t**ub
25.	**ṭh** - as in ligh**t-h**eart	30.	**th** - as in ligh**t-h**eart
26.	**ḍ** - as in **d**ove	31.	**d** – **d**ove
27.	**ḍh** - as in re**d-h**ot	32.	**dh** - as in re**d-h**ot
28.	**ṅ** - as in si**ng**	33.	**n** - as in **n**ut

Sr.no	Labials (pronounced with the lips)	Sr.no	Semivowels
34.	p - pine	39.	y - as in yes
35.	**ph** - as in up-**h**ill	40.	**r** - as in **r**un
36.	**b** - as in **b**ird	41.	**l** - as in **l**ight
37.	**bh** - as in ru**b-h**ard	42.	**v** - as in vine, except when preceded in the same syllable by the consonant, then as in swan
38.	**m** - as in **m**other		

Sr.no	Sibilants	Sr.no	Aspirate
43.	**ś** - as in the German word sprechen	46.	**h** - as in **h**ome
44.	**ṣ** - as in **sh**ine		
45.	**s** - as in **s**un		

Sr.no	Anusvara	Sr.no.	Visarga
47.	**ṁ** - a resonant nasal sound as in the French word bon	48.	**ḥ** - a final h-sound: **aḥ** is pronounced like **aha**; **iḥ** like **ihi**.

There is no strong accentuation of syllables in Sanskrit, or pausing between words in a line, only a flowing of short and long syllables (the long twice as long as the short). A long syllable is one whose vowel is long **(ā, ī, ū, ṛ, e, ai, o, au)** or whose short vowels followed by more than one consonant. The letters ḥ and ṁ count as consonants. Aspirated consonant (consonants followed by an **h)** count as single consonants.

(1) In the throat

ka kha ga gha ṅa ha

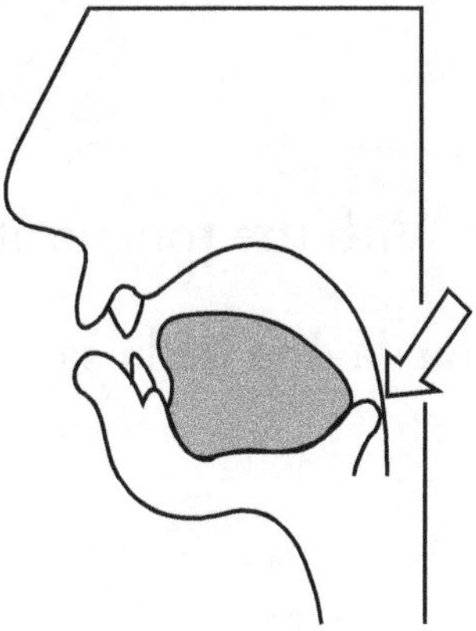

(2) With the tongue
at the rear of the palate

ca cha ja jha ña ya śa

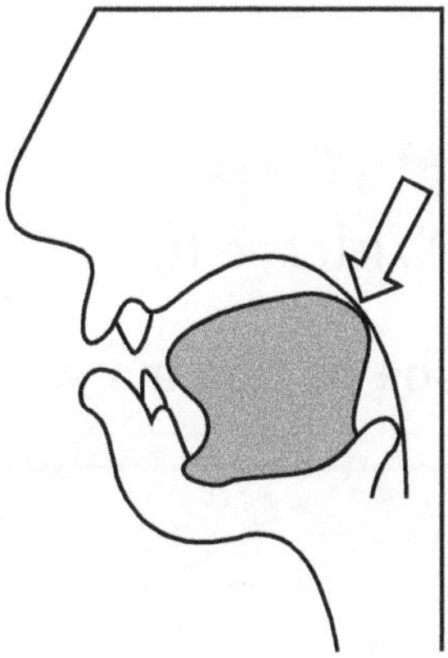

(3) With the tongue
at the top of the palate

ṭa ṭha ḍa ḍha ṇa ra ṣa

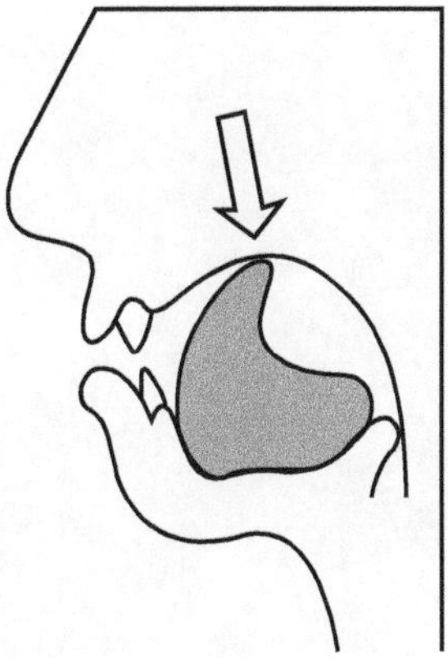

(4) With the tongue at the teeth

ta ha da dha na la sa

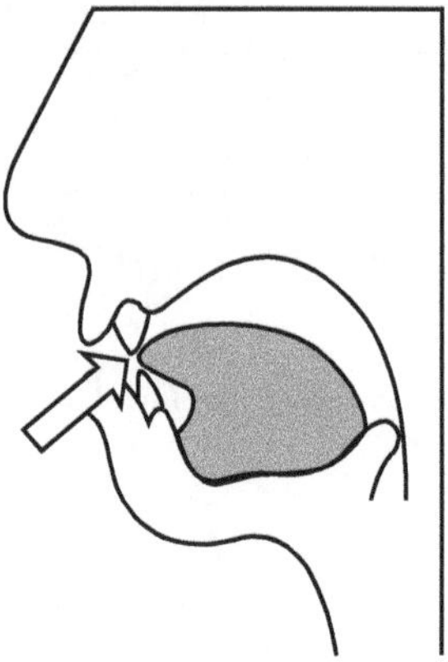

(5) With the lips

pa pha ba bha ma va

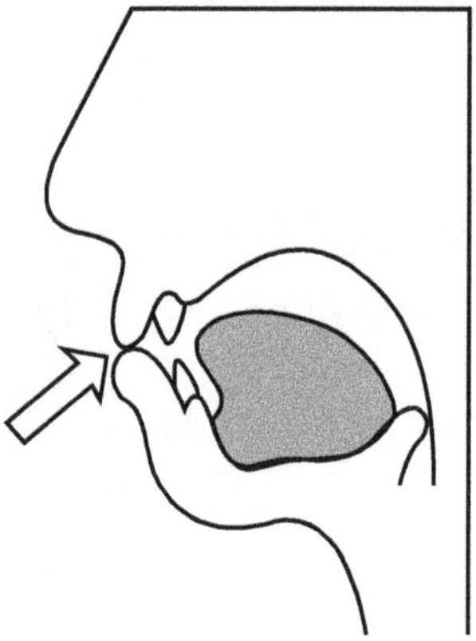

Biography of A.C. Bhaktivedanta Swami Prabhupada

His Divine Grace A. C. Bhaktivedanta Swami Prabhupada was born in 1896 in Calcutta, India. He first met his spiritual master, Srila Bhaktisiddhanta Sarasvati Gosvami, in Calcutta in 1922. Bhaktisiddhanta Sarasvati, a prominent devotional scholar and the founder of sixty-four branches of Gaudiya Mathas (Vedic institutes), liked this educated young man and convinced him to dedicate his life to teaching Vedic knowledge in the Western world. *Śrīla Prabhupāda* became his student, and eleven years later (1933) at Allahabad, he became his formally initiated disciple.

At their first meeting, in 1922, Srila Bhaktisiddhanta Sarasvati Thakura requested *Śrīla Prabhupāda* to broadcast Vedic knowledge through the English language. In the years that followed, *Śrīla Prabhupāda* wrote a commentary on the Bhagavad-gita and in 1944, without assistance, started an English fortnightly magazine.

Recognizing *Śrīla Prabhupāda*'s philosophical learning and devotion, the Gaudiya Vaisnava Society honored him in 1947 with the title "Bhaktivedanta." In 1950, at the age of fifty-four, *Śrīla Prabhupāda* retired from married life, and four years later he adopted the vanaprastha (retired) order to devote more time to his studies and writing. *Śrīla Prabhupāda* traveled to the holy city of Vrndavan, where he lived in very humble circumstances in the historic medieval temple of Radha-Damodara. There he engaged for several years in deep study and writing. He accepted the renounced order of life (sannyasa) in 1959. At Radha-Damodara, *Śrīla Prabhupāda* began work on his life's masterpiece: a multivolume translation and commentary on the 18,000-verse Srimad-Bhagavatam (*Bhagavata Purana*). He also wrote *Easy Journey to Other Planets*.

After publishing three volumes of Bhagavatam, *Śrīla Prabhupāda* came to the United States, in 1965, to fulfill the mission of his spiritual master. Since that time, His Divine Grace has written over sixty volumes of authoritative translations, commentaries and summary studies of the philosophical and religious classics of India.

In 1965, when he first arrived by freighter in New York City, *Śrīla Prabhupāda* was practically penniless. It was after almost a year of great difficulty that he established the International Society for Krishna Consciousness in July of 1966. Under his careful guidance, the Society has grew within a decade to a worldwide confederation of almost one hundred asramas, schools, temples, institutes and farm communities.

In 1968, *Śrīla Prabhupāda* created New Vrndavan, an experimental Vedic community in the hills of West Virginia. Inspired by the success of New Vrndavan, then a thriving farm community of more than one thousand acres, his students founded several similar communities in the United States and abroad.

In 1972, His Divine Grace introduced the Vedic system of primary and secondary education in the West by founding the Gurukula school in Dallas, Texas. The school began with three children in 1972, and by the beginning of 1975 the enrollment had grown to one hundred fifty.

Śrīla Prabhupāda also inspired the construction of a large international center at Sridhama Mayapur in West Bengal, India, which is also the site for a planned Institute of Vedic Studies. A similar project is the magnificent Krsna-Balarama Temple and International Guest House in Vrndavana, India. These are centers where Westerners can live to gain firsthand experience of Vedic culture.

Śrīla Prabhupāda's most significant contribution, however, is his books. Highly respected by the academic community for their authoritativeness, depth and clarity, they are used as standard textbooks in numerous college courses. His writings have been translated into eleven languages. The Bhaktivedanta Book Trust, established in 1972 exclusively to publish the works of His Divine Grace, has thus become the world's largest publisher of books in the field of Indian religion and philosophy.

In the last ten years of his life, in spite of his advanced age, *Śrīla Prabhupāda* circled the globe twelve times on lecture tours that have took him to six continents. In spite of such a vigorous schedule, *Śrīla Prabhupāda* continued to write prolifically. His writings constitute a veritable library of Vedic philosophy, religion, literature and culture.

Śrīla Prabhupāda left us a veritable library of Vedic philosophy and culture. Highly respected by scholars for their authority, depth, and clarity, his books are used at colleges and universities around the world.

The Bhaktivedanta Book Trust publishes his works in over 50 languages.

Find out more about the kind and compassionate person that *Śrīla Prabhupāda* was, and how he was able to change so many lives and accomplish so much in such a short time.

Biography of the Author

The author was born as Philip Burbank in 1949, in Brooklyn, New York. In January 1969, while studying at the University at Buffalo, he joined ISKCON and the same year was initiated by A. C. Bhaktivedanta Swami Prabhupāda, receiving the name Prahlādānanda Dāsa. In 1975 he joined the Rādhā-Damodara preaching bus tour, organized by Tamäl Kṛṣṇa Goswami and Vishnujana Swami. In 1982 he took sannyasa and in 1986 he became one of the initiating gurus in ISKCON. In 1989 he became a member the Vrindavan Institute for Higher Education, and gave monthly seminars on Ayurveda and other topics twice a year for 7 years. In 1990 he was appointed to head the Governing Body Commission's Ministry of Health and Welfare. In 1991, the GBC also appointed him the head of Sannyāsa Ministry.

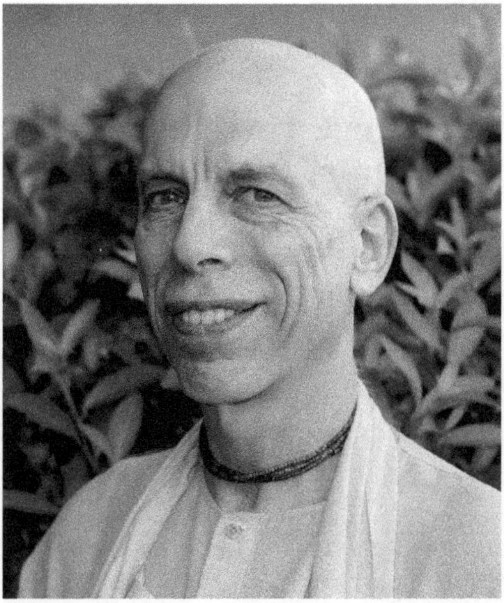

Glossary

Annakūṭa ceremony—a ceremony where the Deity is worshiped by large offering of food.

Ārati—a ceremony in which one greets and worships the Lord in the Deity form of the Supreme Personality of Godhead by offering Him things such as incense and a flame from a lamp with ghee-soaked wicks.

Arjuna—an intimate friend of Lord Kṛṣṇa.

Āsana—seat, or throne; a sitting posture in yoga practice.

Aśvinī-kumāras—Expert Āyurvedic physicians on the higher planetary systems

Āyurveda—the section of the Vedas which expounds the Vedic science of medicine delivered by Lord Dhanvantari, the incarnation of the Supreme Lord as a physician.

Balarāma (Baladeva)—the first plenary expansion of the Supreme Personality of Godhead, Lord Kṛṣṇa.

Bali Māhāraja—the king of the demons who gave three paces of land to Vamanadeva, the dwarf incarnation of Lord Viṣṇu, and thereby became a great devotee by surrendering everything to Him.

Bhagavad-gītā—a seven-hundred verse record of a conversation between

Lord Kṛṣṇa and His disciple, Arjuna, from the Bhīṣma Parva of the Mahābhārata of Vedavyāsa. It contains the essence of all Vedic wisdom.

Bhakti-yoga—The process of devotional service to the Supreme Personality of Godhead, Lord Kṛṣṇa.

Bhaktisiddhānta—Sarasvatī Ṭhākura Gosvāmī Mahārāja Prabhupāda (1874–1937) the spiritual master of His Divine Grace A. C. Bhaktivedanta Swami Prabhupāda, and thus the spiritual grandfather of the present day Kṛṣṇa consciousness movement.

Bhaktivinoda Ṭhākura (1838–1915)—the great-grandfather of the present-day Kṛṣṇa consciousness movement, the spiritual master of Śrīla Gaura-kiśora dāsa Bābājī, the father of Śrila Bhaktisiddhānta Sarasvatī, and the grand-spiritual master of His Divine Grace A. C. Bhaktivedanta Swami Prabhupāda.

Bharata Mahārāja—an ancient king of India and a great devotee of the Lord from whom the Pāṇḍavas descended.

Bhīṣmadeva—the grandfather of the Pāṇḍavas, and the most powerful and venerable warrior on the Battlefield of Kurukṣetra.

Brahmā—The principal demigod who assists Lord Krishna by engineering the universe

Brāhmaṇa—One of the four orders of occupational life, *brāhmaṇa*, *kṣatriya*, *vaiśya* and *śūdra*. The brāhmaṇas are the intellectual class and their occupation is hearing Vedic literature, teaching Vedic literature, learning deity worship and teaching deity worship, receiving charity and giving charity.

Brahmacarya—celibate student life; the first order of Vedic spiritual life; the vow of strict abstinence from sex indulgence.

Caitanya-bhāgavata—Early biography of Lord Caitanya Mahāprabhu.

Caitanya Mahāprabhu, (1486–1534)—Lord Kṛṣṇa in the aspect of His own devotee. He appeared in Navadvīpa, West Bengal, and inaugurated the congregational chanting of the holy names of the Lord to teach pure love of God by means of *saṅkīrtana.*

Cyavana Muni—Ancient sage.

Darśana—the act of seeing and being seen by the Deity in the temple or by a spiritually advanced person.

Deity—A form of God as represented in stone, metal, wood, or as a painted picture, through which He accepts the service of His devotees.

Demigods—universal controllers and residents of the higher planets. They are conditioned souls who the Supreme Lord empowers to represent Him in the management of the universe.

Dhanvantari—the incarnation of the Supreme Lord who is the father of medical science.

Divya-jñāna—Spiritual knowledge.

Gaṅgā Sāgara melā—Spiritual festival periodically performed near sacred rivers such as the Ganges.

GBC—A body of managers that *Śrīla Prabhupāda* appointed to oversee the activities of ISKCON.

God-brother (sister)—Those who are initiated by the same spiritual master.

Gosvāmī—a person who has his senses under full control: the title of a person in the renounced order of life, *sannyasa.* (*go*–senses + *svamī*-master) master of the senses.

Gṛhastha—householder stage of life. One who lives in God conscious married life and raises a family in Kṛṣṇa consciousness; regulated householder living according to the Vedic social system; the second order of Vedic spiritual life.

Guru Mahārāja—A respectful way of addressing one's spiritual master.

Gurukula—a school of Vedic learning. Boys begin at five years old and live as celibate students, guided by a spiritual master.

Hare Kṛṣṇa mantra—a sixteen-word prayer composed of the names Hare, Kṛṣṇa, and Rāma: Hare Kṛṣṇa, Hare Kṛṣṇa, Kṛṣṇa Kṛṣṇa, Hare Hare, Hare Rāma, Hare Rāma, Rāma Rāma, Hare Hare. Hare is the personal form of God's own happiness, His eternal consort, Śrīmatī Rādhārāṇī. Kṛṣṇa, "the all-attractive one," and Rāma, "the all-pleasing one," are names of God.

Hiraṇyakaśipu—a powerful demon and great atheist who tormented his son Prahlāda Mahārāja, a great devotee, and was killed by Kṛṣṇa in His incarnation as Nṛsiṁhadeva (the half man-half lion form of Lord Viṣṇu).

His Divine Grace—One who represents the mercy potency of the Supreme Lord.

Indra—the chief demigod of heaven and presiding deity of rain, and the father of Arjuna. He is the son of Aditi.

Initiation—Formally taking spiritual vows.

Japa—the soft recitation of the Kṛṣṇa's holy names as a private meditation, with the aid of 108 prayer beads.

Jīva Gosvāmī—one of the Six Gosvāmīs of Vṛndāvana and the nephew of Rupa and Sanātana Gosvāmīs.

Juhu Beach—A beach in Mumbai.

Kali-yuga—the "Age of Quarrel and Hypocrisy" The fourth and last age in the cycle of a *mahā-yuga*. This is the present age in which we are now living. It began 5,000 years ago and lasts for a total of 432,000 years. It is characterized by irreligious practice and stringent material miseries.

Kardama Muni—An ancient sage and *yogi*.

Kīrtana—Narrating or singing the glories of the Supreme Personality of Godhead and His Holy Names.

Kṛṣṇa consciousness—To be aware of Lord Kṛṣṇa.

Krishna consciousness movement—The movement meant to help revive people's original consciousness of the Supreme Lord, Lord Kṛṣṇa.

Kṣatriya—third of the four orders of the *varṇāśrama* system. A warrior who is inclined to fight and lead others. The administrative or protective occupation according to the system of four social and spiritual orders.

Kubja—A prostitute who became a devotee of Lord Kṛṣṇa.

Mahārāja—king, ruler, sannyasi (renounced order of life)

Maṅgala-arati—the daily predawn worship ceremony honoring the Deity of the Supreme Lord.

Māyā-śakti—Māyā–illusion; an energy of Krṣna's which deludes the living entity into forgetfulness of the Supreme Lord. That which is not, unreality, deception, forgetfulness, material illusion.

Murāri Caitanya dāsa—A pure devotee in Lord Caitanya's pastimes.

Murāri Gupta—A doctor and pure devotee of Lord Caitanya.

Names for the Supreme Lord (God): Absolute Truth, Vishnu, Godhead, Supersoul, Krsna, Rama.

Nārada Muni—a pure devotee of the Lord, one of the sons of Lord

Brahmā, who travels throughout the universes in his eternal body, glorifying devotional service while delivering the science of bhakti.

New Vrindaban—An ISKCON temple and spiritual retreat in West Virginia, USA.

Śeṣa Nāga—an expansion of Lord Balarāma or Saṅkarṣaṇa who takes the form of a many-hooded serpent and serves as Lord Viṣṇu's couch and other paraphernalia.

Prabhupāda, Śrīla—Śrīla Prabhupāda (1896-1977) His Divine Grace A. C. Bhaktivedanta Swami Prabhupāda. He is the tenth generation from Caitanya Mahāprabhu. The founder-*ācārya*, spiritual master of the International Society for Krishna Consciousness (ISKCON).

Prabhupāda—master at whose feet all other masters surrender.

Prahlāda Maharāja—a great devotee of Lord Kṛṣṇa who was persecuted by his atheistic father, Hiraṇyakaśipu, but was always protected by the Lord and ultimately saved by the Lord in the form of Nṛsiṁhadeva.

Prasāda, or prasādam—"the mercy of Lord Kṛṣṇa." Food prepared for the pleasure of Kṛṣṇa and offered to Him with love and devotion.

Raghunātha dāsa Gosvāmī—one of the Six Gosvāmīs of Vṛndāvana.

Rounds—Number of times one chants the Hare Krsna maha-mantra around a string of beads.

Rules and regulations—Activities that should and should not be done according to the scriptures.

Sādhu—a saint or Krishna conscious devotee, or Vaiṣṇava.

Saṅkīrtana—The congregational glorification of the Lord through chanting His holy name.

Sanskrit—the oldest language in the world.
Sanātana Gosvāmī—one of the Six Gosvāmīs of Vṛndāvana who was authorized by Lord Caitanya Mahāprabhu to establish and distribute the philosophy of Kṛṣṇa consciousness.

Sannyāsa—the renounced order, and fourth stage of Vedic spiritual life in the Vedic system of *varṇāsrama*-dharma, which is free from family relationships and in which all activities are completely dedicated to self-realization.

Sannyāsī—one in the *sannyāsa* (renounced) order.

Sāraṅga Ṭhākura—A great devotee of Lord Caitanya.

Shajiya—One who takes spiritual life cheaply and doesn't follow strictly the rules and regulations as given in the scriptures.

Śrīmad Bhāgavatam—A scripture of eighteen thousand verses compiled by Vyasadeva.

Srīvāsa Ṭhākura—the incarnation of Śri Nārada Muni in Lord Caitanya's pastimes.

Śūdra—a member of the fourth social order, laborer class, in the traditional Vedic social system.

Sukadeva Gosvāmī—an exhalted devotee who recited the *Śrīmad-Bhāgavatam* to King Parīkṣit during the last seven days of the King's life.

Śukrācārya—the spiritual master of the demons.

Svāyambhuva Manu—the Manu who appears first in Brahmā's day and who was the grandfather of Dhruva Mahārāja.

Tilaka—sacred clay markings placed on the forehead and other parts of the body to designate one as a follower of Viṣṇu, Rāma, Śiva, Vedic culture, etc.

Uddhava—a learned disciple of Bṛhaspati and confidential friend of Lord Kṛṣṇa in Dvārakā.

Ugra-karma—evil activities.

Upavāsa—fasting

Vaiṣṇava—a devotee of the Supreme Lord, Viṣṇu, or Kṛṣṇa.

Vaiśya (Vaishyas)—member of the mercantile or agricultural class, according to the system of four social orders and four spiritual orders.

Vānaprastha—retired family life, in which one quits home to cultivate renunciation and travels from holy place to holy place in preparation for the renounced order of life; the third order of Vedic spiritual life; a retired householder.

Vedic—pertaining to a culture in which all aspects of human life are under the guidance of the Vedas.

Vṛndāvana—Kṛṣṇa's eternal abode, where He fully manifests His quality of sweetness; the village on this earth in which He enacted His childhood pastimes five thousand years ago.

Vyāsadeva (Vyāsa)—the literary incarnation of God, and the greatest philosopher of ancient times.

Yamarāja—the demigod of death, who passes judgment on non-devotees at the time of death. He is the son of the sun-god and the goddess of the sacred river Yamunā.

Yamunā—the sacred river where Kṛṣṇa performed many pastimes.

Yukta-vairāgya—befitting, real renunciation, in which one utilizes everything in the service of the Supreme Lord.

Bibliography

Bhagavad-gītā As It Is, Bhaktivedanta Swami Prabhupāda, A. C., Los Angeles: Bhaktivedanta Book Trust, 1983.

Conversations with Śrīla Prabhupaāda, Bhaktivedanta Swami Prabhupāda, A. C., Sandy Ridge, NC: Bhaktivedanta Archives.

Govinda Swami, B. B.

Great Transcendental Adventure, Dāsa, Kūrma, Australia: Chakra Press, 1999.

"Interview with Nanda Kumar dāsa," Dāsa, Nanda Kumar

Kṛṣṇa: the Supreme Personality of Godhead, Bhaktivedanta Swami Prabhupāda, A. C., Los Angeles: Bhaktivedanta Book Trust, 1970.

Life with the Perfect Master, Gosvāmī, Satsvarūpa Dāsa, Port Royal, PA: Gita Nagari Press, 1983.

My *Glorious Master,* Dāsa, Bhūrijana, Vrindavan: VIHE Publications, 1996.

The Nectar of Devotion, Bhaktivedanta Swami Prabhupāda, A. C., New York: Bhaktivedanta Book Trust, 1979.

Nectar of Instruction, Rūpa Gosvāmī, translation and purports by

Bhaktivedanta Swami Prabhupāda, A. C., Los Angeles: Bhaktivedanta Book Trust, 1975.

Perfect Questions, Perfect Answers, Bhaktivedanta Swami Prabhupāda, A. C., Los Angeles: Bhaktivedanta Book Trust, 1977.

Prabhupāda Nectar, Gosvāmī, Satsvarūpa Dāsa, Port Royal, PA: GN Press, 1995.

Raāja-vidyaā, the King of Knowledge, Bhaktivedanta Swami Prabhupāda, A. C., Los Angeles: Bhaktivedanta Book Trust, 1975.

The Science of Self-Realization, Bhaktivedanta Swami Prabhupāda, A. C., Los Angeles: Bhaktivedanta Book Trust, 1977.

"Remembrance by Badri Nārāyaṇa dāsa," Dāsa, Badri Nārāyaṇa

Śrī Caitanya-caritaāmṛta, Kṛṣṇadāsa Kavirāja Gosvāmī, translation and purports by Bhaktivedanta Swami Prabhupāda, A. C., Los Angeles: Bhaktivedanta Book Trust, 1996.

Śrī Iśopaniṣad, Bhaktivedanta Swami Prabhupāda, A. C., Los Angeles: Bhaktivedanta Book Trust, 1993.

Śrīlā Prabhupāda Letters, Bhaktivedanta Swami Prabhupāda, Sandy Ridge, NC: Bhaktivedanta Archives.

Srīmad-Bhāgavatam, Bhaktivedanta Swami Prabhupāda, A. C., and his disciples, Los Angeles: Bhaktivedanta Book Trust, 1972–1989.

Śrīlā Prabhupāda-līlāmṛta, Gosvāmī, Satsvarūpa Dāsa, Port Royal, PA: GN Press, 1980.

Transcendental Diary (Volumes 1–5), Dāsa, Hari Śauri, HS Books, 1992–2005.

Acknowledgements

For the English edition of this book, I would like to first thank those who over the years have edited my articles on health: Dravida dasa, Tattvavit dasa, Jaya Bhadra devi dasi, Rupa Sanatana dasa (JDS), and Kancana-valli devi dasi (SRS).

The excerpts from Srila Prabhupada-lilamrta, by Satsvarupa dasa Goswami, and A Transcendental Diary, by Hauri Sauri Prabhu, hopefully have made the book more interesting.

My appreciation goes to Drdha Vrata dasa, who made the arrangements for the cover and the layout, which was done by Mani deep dasa. Yugalakisora dasa (PAS), Omkara dasa (PAS), Damodara dasa (PAS), and Bhakti Prabhava Swami looked over Srila Prabhupada's instructions and gave valuable suggestions.

My yoga teachers, such as Krodhasamani devi dasi and Jose Maria, gave me valuable lessons on health.

Vasant Lad, Rama Prasad, and Raga Manjari devi dasi, and Liladhara Gupta from Vrindavan have given me many insights into Ayurveda.

Mrtyuhara Prabhu deserves special appreciation for donating the printing costs of the book.

CPSIA information can be obtained
at www.ICGtesting.com
Printed in the USA
LVHW031154141019
634125LV00002B/333/P

9 781723 167584